Health in Saudi Arabia

Vol. Two

Health in Saudi Arabia

Vol. Two

2nd Edition

ZOHAIR A. SEBAI

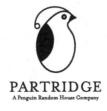

PARTRIDGE

A Penguin Random House Company

To order additional copies of this book, contact
Toll Free 800 101 2657 (Singapore)
Toll Free 1 800 81 7340 (Malaysia)
orders.singapore@partridgepublishing.com

www.partridgepublishing.com/singapore

CONTENTS

PREFACE

Health in Saudi Arabia, Volume I, published in 1985, presented an introduction to health problems, health manpower and medical education in Saudi Arabia.

Volume II now discusses the epidemiology of certain health problems and the development of health services and health manpower. The material in Volume II is based upon a two-year project supported by **King Abdul Aziz City for Science and Technology** under Grant No. AT-5-26.

The two volumes cannot be comprehensive, but strive to give baseline information on health in a country which is developing very fast but still is relatively inexperienced in medical research.

The first edition of the book has been published in the year 1987. Still it would be of interest for those who would like to study health and health services development in the country.

ACKNOWLEDGEMENT

I wish to thank the members of the editorial committee, Professors David A. Price Evans, Sheikh Mahjoob, Hassan Abu Aisha and Hassan Bahakim, and Dr Monir Madkour for their critical reviews and constructive ideas.

I am also grateful to Dr Othman Rabia and Mr. Adnan Al-Beshr for supervising the fieldwork, Dr Adnan Barri for the data analysis and Dr Hassan Bella for preparing the educational material. The great assistance given by Mr. Abdul Rashid Bhatti in typing the manuscript on the word processor, Mr. Eddie Musngi in typesetting and composing, Mrs. Hoda Sharabash and Mrs. Jane Duncan in reviewing and editing, made the writing a pleasant task.

بسم الله الرحمن الرحيم

مقدمــــة

بين يدي القارىء الكريم الجزء الثاني من كتاب الصحة في المملكة العربية السعودية، وهو موجه إلى الأطباء وطلبة الطب والدراسات الطبية العليا، وإلى جميع المهتمين بالتعليم الطبي والخدمات الصحية. نرجو أن يسد الكتاب بعض الفراغ الذي نجده في المعلومات الصحية في بلادنا.

استعرضنا في الجزء الأول، الذي صدر في مطلع عام ١٤٠٥هـ، بعض المشاكل الصحية في المجتمعات الريفية والبدوية، مثل تربة البقوم وقرى خليص وعسير وغامد وزهران وجيزان، كما استعرضنا قضية التعليم الطبي وجوانب من الخدمات الصحية.

وفي الجزء الثاني الذي هو بين يديك، سوف نكمل ما بدأناه من بحث، وقد قسمناه إلى قسمين، يتناول القسم الأول المشاكل الصحية، بينا يتناول القسم الثاني الخدمات الصحية.

في القسم الأول، استعرضنا عشر مشاكل صحية رئيسية في بلادنا.. هي الملاريا والبلهارسيا والتهاب الكبد الفيروسي والتراخوما والسل وأمراض التغذية ومرض السكر وأمراض السرطان وأمراض هيموجلوبين الدم وحوادث الطرق.. تطرقنا إلى كل منها من حيث حجم المشكلة ومدى انتشارها وأكثر فئات السكان تعرضاً للإصابة بها، إلى جانب العوامل البيئية والاجتماعية التي تصاحبها وتساعد على انتشارها. واختتمنا كل فصل من الفصول العشرة بمجمل عن طرق الوقاية من المشكلة ومكافحتها. ولو كان هناك متسع من الوقت، لاستعرضنا مشاكل أخرى، بالإضافة إلى ما استعرضناه مثل حمى مالطا ومرض الليشمانيا وأمراض القلب الروماتزمية ومشكلة الصحة في مواسم الحج، وهي مشاكل مهمة تستحق أن تدرس. ولعلنا نستطيع أن نتحدث عنها في كتاب لاحق، أو قد يتصدى لها ولغيرها بعض الزملاء الباحثين.

تطرقنا في القسم الثاني من الكتاب، إلى الخدمات الصحية بالمملكة وركزنا على جانبين أساسيين، هما الرعاية الصحية الأولية، والقوى البشرية العاملة في القطاع الصحي. تحدثنا عن التطور السريع الذي حظيت به الرعاية الصحية في المملكة، وألممنا بمفهوم الرعاية الصحية كما تبنته دول العالم الأعضاء في هيئة الصحة العالمية، وعرجنا من ذلك على طرق تطبيق الرعاية الصحية في المملكة ووسائل تطويرها. وفي معرض الحديث عن القوى البشرية استعرضنا جوانب من التعليم الطبي في المملكة ومدى ملاءمته للخدمات الصحية المطلوبة، وانتهينا إلى وضع بعض المقترحات لتطوير القوى البشرية في المملكة كماً وكيفاً.

10

والنتيجة التي نخلص منها بعد قراءة الكتاب هي أن مستقبل الرعاية الصحية في بلادنا يعتمد أولاً على عداد الفريق الطبي المتكامل إعداداً يتلاءم مع طبيعة المشاكل الصحية الحالية والمتوقعة مستقبلاً، ثانياً عطاء الجوانب الوقائية حقها من الاهتمام جنباً إلى جنب مع العلاج، ثالثاً تطوير الرعاية الصحية الأولية. وإني لأرجو من الله أن يوفقني إلى تعريب الكتاب حتى يكون في متناول يد القارىء باللغة العربية. وأن يجعل في الكتاب بعض الفائدة للأطباء والدارسين في كليات الطب وطلبة الدراسات العليا والقائمين على أمور الصحة في بلادنا.

وفي النهاية، أحب أن أتقدم بالشكر الجزيل إلى ولاة الأمر في بلادنا على تشجيعهم للبحث العلمي ورعايتهم للباحثين، وأتمنى من الله أن يزدهم توفيقاً فيما يصبون إليه من خير لهذه الأمة. وأقدر للمسئولين في مدينة الملك عبد العزيز للبحوث والتكنولوجيا قيامهم بتمويل الدراسة التي تمخض عنها هذا الكتاب والتي استغرقت نحواً من سنتين. كما أشكر المسئولين في وزارة الصحة على مشاركتهم في العمل الحقلي الذي قام على أساسه جزء كبير من الدراسة. وإلى جميع الإخوة والزملاء الذين شاركوا في قراءة ومناقشة مسودات الكتاب وإلى الذين قاموا على إخراجه وطباعته أقدم شكري وامتناني.

و بالله التوفيق

زهــيـر أحـمـد السباعي

INTRODUCTION

During the last decade Saudi Arabia has experienced a rapid development which is probably unsurpassed by any other nation. It has been a historical phenomenon. The government revenues from oil and other sources recorded an almost 40-fold increase, rising from SR5.7 billion in 1970 to SR211 billion in 1980 (US$ 1 equals SR 3.75). In the same period of time the total number of schools increased from 3,100 to more than 11,000, representing an average growth of 14.5%. From 1970 to 1985, the number of hospital beds increased from 9,039 to 30,707 and the number of physicians increased from 1,172 to 14,335. The natural population growth is estimated at 2.8% per year.

The expansion of health services has brought medical care to almost every village in the country. The rapid growth in economy, health care facilities, urbanization and mass media have changed, in one way or another, health knowledge and the attitudes and practices of the people.

In spite of the dramatic development in the health sector, some problems remain. The physical development has not been complemented in this short period of time by a parallel development in national human resources. The expatriate health personnel face cultural and language barriers, especially in rural areas. Information on the magnitude and distribution of health problems and resources is sporadic and incomplete.

Health services remain predominantly curative. Most of the health personnel are products of patient-oriented, hospital-based medical institutes, and the people's demand, as expected, is for curative care.

This volume discusses certain health problems, mostly from an epidemiological perspective, and presents the main features of the health services and health manpower in Saudi Arabia.

The problems of malaria, schistosomiasis, tuberculosis, viral hepatitis, trachoma, nutritional disorders, diabetes, disorders of hemoglobin synthesis, cancer and road traffic injuries are discussed. The selection of these problems was made partly because of their importance and partly because they are within my field of interest. Other problems such as cardiovascular diseases, leishmaniasis and health during pilgrimage would also have been discussed if time had permitted.

The chapter on health services and health manpower is based on a field survey carried out under the auspices of the Department of Medical Planning and Research, Ministry of Health, with a contribution from the Department of Statistics, College of Sciences, King Saud University. The voluminous data which came out of the survey are under analysis by the Ministry of Health and College of Sciences. I used just some of the data, relevant to the purpose, in the book.

Volumes I and II of **Health in Saudi Arabia** have been written for physician medical students and health personnel in general. I hope that they will provide the reader with basic knowledge of health in Saudi Arabia and will stimulate discussion and bring new ideas.

ZOHAIR SEBAI

CHAPTER I

HEALTH PROBLEMS

Health problems in Saudi Arabia vary from communicable diseases such as hepatitis and schistosomiasis, to those of a modern society with stress related diseases, pollution and traffic injuries. In this chapter ten selected health problems will be discussed.

- Malaria
- Schistosomiasis
- Tuberculosis
- Viral Hepatitis
- Trachoma
- Nutritional Disorders
- Diabetes
- Hemoglobin Synthesis Disorders
- Cancer
- Road Traffic Injuries

MALARIA

INTRODUCTION

Of all the infectious diseases, malaria has caused the greatest harm to the greatest number of people. Approximately 1.6 billion people live in malarious areas in the tropics and subtropics, and at least 150 million people are infected. One million deaths occur annually in Africa alone.

Man is the only important reservoir of malaria, and the female Anopheles mosquito is the intermediate host. Four *Plasmodium* species cause malaria in man, *P. falciparum* (the malignant form), *P. vivax*, *P. malariae* and *P. ovale*. The clinical picture includes fever, chills, sweating, anaemia and splenic enlargement. Complications, mainly due to the malignant form, can lead to shock, renal failure, jaundice, severe anaemia and coma.

Malaria is a classic example of a disease which must be prevented and not merely treated.

HISTORY

Malaria or Humma al thuluth (the fever which attacks man every third day) has been mentioned in Arabic writings since the pre-Islamic era. In recent times many travellers in the Arabian peninsula including Doughty,[1] Philby [2] and Scott [3] have mentioned malaria as a prevailing disease in Arabia. In the

1948 Marett[4] reported that Anopheles mosquitoes were abundant about the wells and marshy areas in Al-Hasa and Qatif oases and nearly 100% of the population had suffered from malaria at one time or another.

The first reliable data on malaria in Saudi Arabia came from Aramco (Arabian American Oil Company) in the Eastern Province in 1941.[5] Malaria was persistently the most significant health hazard and the leading cause of morbidity and mortality among the Aramco Saudi population. Annual morbidity rates during the period 1941-1947 varied between 1000 and 2700 cases per 10,000. Most of the cases came from the two major oases, Al-Hasa and Qatif and were typical "oasis malaria" described by, Daggy[6] as follows:

"Oasis malaria is characterized by its sharp delimitation to the island-like cultivated areas in a sea of sand. The population is chiefly concentrated in one or two main centers, and the remainder is in scattered small villages surrounded by irrigated date-palm groves. Within this area are also concentrated the breeding places of the anopheline vectors, primarily *Anopheles stephena*. Hence man, mosquito, and parasite are all closely confined to the cultivated areas, and here malaria is hyperendemic. Only a few miles from the well-defined borders of these oases, Bedouins or other travelers are perfectly safe from the disease."

The survey conducted in Qatif in 1947 showed an infant parasite rate of 100%; among other age groups the parasite rate was 85% and the spleen rate in the 2-14 year age group was 93%. Although *P. falciparum, P. vivax*, and *P. malariae* were present, *P. falciparum* was the most important in terms in prevalence, morbidity and mortality.[7]

In 1948 Aramco, with the cooperation of the Ministry of Health, launched the first campaign against malaria and a dramatic reduction in malaria incidence was accomplished by the early 1950s. Cases of anopheline resistance anti-larval measures and the spraying of houses with DDT were recorded.[8] During the 1960s malaria continued to occur in Al-Hasa and Qatif at a lesser rate. In the mid-1970s malaria transmission was completely interrupted and the improvement was well maintained in the Eastern Province[10] (Table 1???

Haemoglobin S, an important gene marker for Al-Hasa and Qatif population gave some protection against *P. falciparum* by reducing the parasite burden affected children.[11]

Preliminary surveys conducted by the Ministry of Health in the early 1950s revealed the endemicity of the disease in many parts of the Kingdom ranging from mesoendemic levels in the Northern and Western Provinces hyperendemic levels in the South Western Provinces. A malariometric survey carried out among children from 2 to 9 years old in Wadi Fatima, near Makkah showed a spleen rate of 32% and a parasite rate of 9%. *Plasmodium falciparum* was the predominent species, and *Anopheles sergenti* and *arabiensis (A. gambiae)* were the main vectors.

The success attained in the Eastern Province encouraged the Ministry of Health in 1952 to initiate a malaria control program assisted by the World Health Organization (WHO) along the route of pilgrims in the Western Province. In 1956, the National Malaria Control Service was created. In 1966, the Ministry of Health signed an agreement with WHO to launch a malaria pre-eradication program. The program paid off. By early 1970 malaria transmission was completely interrupted in the Northern and Western Provinces with the exception of some endemic foci, particularly in Khayber (near Madinah) and the surrounding villages. The South Province was still hyperendemic. In 1970 the pre-eradication program was promoted to control program and action became more progressive.[12]

In the late 1970s, a survey of malaria [13] reported the highest incidence in the Southern region and the lowest from the Northern and Eastern regions. The Western region showed a regular and uniform occurrence of infection throughout the year. Five anopheline vectors were identified; *A. stephemi, A. sergenti, A. gambiae, A. superpictus* and *A. fluriatitis.*

Table 1. Aramco Malaria Incidence by Year and Locale of Acquisition 1964-1970.

Locale of Acquisition	1964	1965	1966	1967	1968	1969	1970	1971	1972	1973	1974
Qatif Oasis	36	182	231	113	25	54	30	12	0	0	0
Al-Hasa Oasis	82	22	14	3	2	1	0	3	0	0	0
Other coastal towns	4	9	6	31	4	2	2	1	0	0	4
Imported	2	7	4	10	32	37	20	24	20	25	45
Total	**124**	**220**	**255**	**157**	**63**	**94**	**52**	**50**	**20**	**25**	**49**

From Ref. 10.

By 1980 malaria was almost under control. Transmission had been interrupted in Qatif, Al Hasa and Sikaka areas, and in the Jeddah, Makkah and Madinah areas malaria had been reduced to a low incidence. In other areas where control measures have not yet, or only partially, been established incidence was rather high. The Tihama area along the Red Sea was left uncovered by the program due to communication difficulties and a shortage of manpower.[12]

In 1981 a malaria training center was established in Jizan and by 1983 eight malaria stations and 15 substations were already established in the Kingdom with the headquarters in Riyadh. By that time malaria control activities had successfully reached all endemic areas in the Kingdom with the exception of Tihama and some residual foci in the Western and South Western provinces.

MANAGEMENT AND ORGANIZATION

The Malaria Control Program is a division of the Department of Preventive Medicine in the Ministry of Health. The headquarters in Riyadh plans and supervises the implementation of the program through eight malaria station and 23 substations distributed all over the country.

The malaria manpower in the headquarters and the peripheral stations is a follows:

public health officers (3), medical officers (18), engineers (12), parasitological technicians (56), entomological technicians (17), field inspectors an supervisors (152), squad leaders (110), and administrators (65).

They face the general problem of health manpower in Saudi Arabia; in that the personnel are mostly non-Saudi, unevenly distributed and require continual training.

The malaria program in the Kingdom is coordinated with the adjacent Arabian countries through committees representing the Ministers of Health of Arabian States of the Gulf Area and North Yemen.[14]

MALARIA IN THE 1980S

Epidemiologically, the country could be divided into three malarious areas (Fig. 1).

1. Areas where malaria transmission has been completely interrupted and the situation is maintained through parasitological and entomological vigilance (Eastern and Northern Provinces).

Figure 1. Malarious areas & main vectors in Saudi Arabia - 1983.

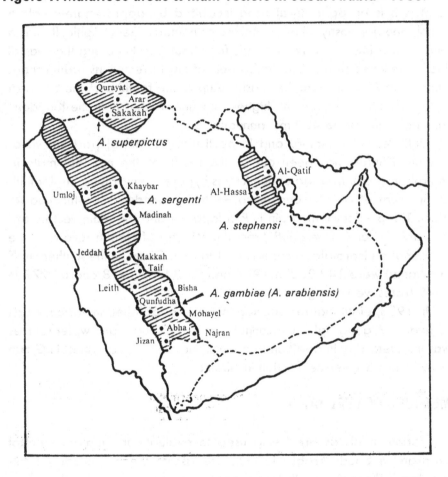

From: Ref. 16.

2. Areas where malaria transmission has been interrupted but residual foci remain (Western Province).
3. Areas where control has been recently initiated (Southern Province).

Tihama presents a special case, being the most endemic area in the country. It is an agricultural area inhabited by approximately half a million people, mostly villagers and some nomads. Geographically it is a long narrow lowland which extends for about 600 km along the coastal line of the Red Sea down to the borders of North Yemen. Its width ranges from 70 to 100 km from the seashore up to the foothills of the Sarawat Mountains. The area has the highest amount of rainfall in the Kingdom, ranging from 300 to 400 mm annually.

Until recently Tihama, and in particular its central part known as Tihamat Kahtan, has been out of the reach of the national malaria control program. Malaria endemicity is hyperendemic along the foothills of Sarawat Mountains and meso — to hypoendemic on the coastal plain. The predominant strain is *P. falciparum* and the main vectors are *A. arabiensis* and *A. serganti*. From the Ministry of Health records,[15] the number of clinical malaria cases reported from Gizan (in the southern half of Tihama) were 142,283 in 1977 and 92,847 in 1978 and 67,277 in 1979 (rates were not given).

In 1983, eight malaria substations were established in various parts of Tihama. A geographical reconnaissance of premises and water sources was initiated. This, in addition to the training center established in Gizan in 1981 has accelerated action in Tihama.

METHODS OF EVALUATION

Various methods are being used to evaluate the malaria control program in Saudi Arabia in order to assess the magnitude of the problem.[16] These include the following.

PASSIVE CASE DETECTION (PCD)

This is the principal parasitological assessment method under current use. All hospitals, health centers and dispensaries are required by law to report every suspected malaria case and send with the report a blood film to the Ministry of Health. Tables 2 and 3 show the results of passive case detection of malaria from all over the Kingdom. Recently there has been an increase in the rate probably due to improved diagnostic methods.

Table 2. Malaria Prevalence: Results of Passive Case Detection from all over the Kingdom 1981-1983.

Year	No. of Reported Cases	No. Positive	% Positive
1981	138,728	4,857	3.5%
1982	249,224	14,325	5.7%
1983	281,566	16,385	5.8%

From Ref. 16.

Table 3. Malaria: Results of PCD in the Provinces, 1983.

Province	No. Examined	No. Positive	% Positive
Eastern and Northern	96,233	673	0.7
Western	58,925	2.412	4.0
Southern	126,408	13,300	10.5
Total	**281,566**	**16,385**	**5.8**

Modified from Ref. 16.

MALARIOMETRIC SURVEY

School children 6-9 years old are examined for an enlarged spleen, and a sample of blood is taken from the finger. These examinations are usually carried out in highly endemic areas in order to measure the prevalence.

INFANT PARASITE SURVEY

In certain villages all babies in the age group of 0-12 months old are examined monthly for blood parasites. This survey measures the incidence and defines the malaria transmission season.

EPIDEMIOLOGICAL CONTACT SURVEY (ECS)

This survey is carried out in hypoendemic or malaria-free areas to detect the source of infection for any positive case found. In the Eastern and Northern Provinces, in 1983, the 16 malaria cases found by ECS were imported. In the Western and Southern provinces the ECS was rather difficult to conduct because of constant movements of the inhabitants.

MASS BLOOD SURVEY (MBS)

Finger blood specimens are taken from inhabitants of new settlement areas (Hejrat) for baseline data.

COMPULSORY BLOOD EXAMINATION OF ARRIVING FOREIGN LABORERS

All laborers coming from malarious countries are tested for blood parasites before being granted work permits.

ENTOMOLOGICAL SURVEYS

Entomological surveys are carried yearly in malarious areas to study the density, distribution, types and behaviour of the vector.

ACTIVE CASE DETECTION (ACD)

This house-to-house survey method was practiced in Qatif and Hassa oases, Eastern province, before the elimination of malaria in the mid-1970s.

Table 4 shows malaria distribution according to parasite species in different regions, as a result of combined examinations by PCD, ECS and MBS conducted in the years 1981-1983.

Table 4. Malaria Distribution According to Species 1983

	Parasite Species %			
	P. falciparum	P. vivax	P. malariae	**Total**
Eastern and Northern	45	29	26	100
Western	50	49	1	100
Southern	96	3	1	100
Total	**87**	**11**	**2**	**100**

From Ref. 17.

CONTROL MEASURES

Since the initiation of the anti-malaria program in 1948, the experience of the country in control measures is much developed. The 1960s showed progress in planning with the help of WHO (WHO malaria experts exceed all other experts in number). An overall success was intermingled with transient periods of failure; all depending on the level of planning, management, supervision, budget allocations and skills of personnel. A major contribution to the success was the accelerated development in the socioeconomic situation and the subsequent improvement in housing, nutrition and education. The relative susceptibilities of man, parasite and vector constantly played an important role.

The control measures have always varied according to the time and place they were carried out but they were, in general, a combination of the following:

HOUSE RESIDUAL SPRAYING WITH DDT

This constitutes the major type of action. (Sorry for the "Silent Spring" in Saudi Arabia!)[17] Its effectiveness depends on the potency of the insecticide, the quality and timing of its application and the acceptance of the local people. The degree of DDT hazard to man is under extensive investigation.[18]

LARVICIDAL OPERATIONS WITH ABATE EMULSION

This aims at reducing the density of the adult mosquitos to a level sufficient to interrupt the transmission of the disease.

WATER MANAGEMENT METHODS

These methods include draining pools, filling pot holes, ditching, removal of algae and aqueous vegetation. They have the advantage of being "natural", but the disadvantage of facing apathy from both health personnel and the general public.

SPRAYING BY ULTRA LOW VOLUME SPRAYING MACHINES

The spray contains a mixture of synthetic pyrethroid insecticides and is used for indoor and outdoor space spraying to treat the suspected and potential resting places of the vector. It always carries the hazard of creating vector resistance if applied indiscriminately, as it is the case in using DDT irrationally.

BIOLOGICAL CONTROL USING LARVIVOROUS FISH

Some trials have been made using this method and it is worth a serious effort.

CHEMOTHERAPY

Since 87% of all confirmed cases of malaria in the country are from *P. falciparum* the general line of treatment is to aim for radical cure; 1500 mg chloroquine and 45 mg primaquine are administered over 3 days to any highly suspected malaria case as well as to microscopically confirmed cases. If the results are positive for *P. vivax* or *P. malariae*, an additional dose of 15 mg primaquine is administered daily for 11 days.

Expatriates coming from Far East countries known to carry the chloroquine-resistant strain of *P. falciparum*, are given 45 mg primaquine regardless of the clinical or laboratory results.

PROBLEMS FACING THE CONTROL PROGRAM

Although the control program has proved generally successful, problems tend to rise from time to time.

IMPORTED/INDUCED MALARIA

People coming from malarious areas abroad or from within the country can always potentially introduce malaria to malaria-free areas when the vector is present. The practice of issuing a certificate of freedom from malaria for pilgrims and expatriate laborers on the basis of a negative blood film is not sufficient since many of them harbor latent parasitemia. The danger of introducing chloroquine-resistant strains of *P. falciparum* in this way from Far Eastern and African countries is always a threat.[19]

OCCASIONAL EPIDEMICS

Even in well maintained areas, epidemics can erupt due to climatic changes. This occurred, for example, in the Western Province in 1950, 1957 and 1982 after heavy rainfalls and floods.

INSUFFICIENT MANAGEMENT

In Mohayal in the Southern Province, for example, the progress made in 1980 was lost in the following years. The parasite rate increased from 4.0% in 1980 to 11.9% in 1983. This occurred because of managerial problems resulting in the reduction of residual spraying and an inadequate coverage by larvicides. The same happened in Qunfudha and Lith.[17]

WHICH WAY FORWARD?

The progress made in the malaria program in Saudi Arabia from the time of its inception in 1948 is possibly one of the most significant achievements in public health in the Kingdom over the last 30 years. The challenge which the country now faces is to control malaria in the Southern Province and in the residual foci in the Western Province, while maintaining the rest of country malaria-free. This could be accomplished by improving the following:

1. Training of malaria personnel;
2. Screening methods for pilgrims and expatriate laborers coming from malarious countries;
3. Administration and evaluation of the program;
4. Active participation of other governmental and non-governmental organizations (including local communities) in the program;
5. Integration of the program with primary health care.

There are still hopes that a multiple vaccine will eventually be developed containing one component that blocks sporozoites or intraerythrocytic stages, and one that blocks transmission through vectors.

REFERENCES

1. **Doughty CM.** *Travels in Arabia deserta.* London: Jonathan Cape, 1921.
2. **Philby H, St. J.** *The Empty Quarter.* London: Methuen, 1933.
3. **Scott H.** *In the High Yemen.* London: Murray, 1942.
4. **Marett WC.** Some medical problems met in Saudi Arabia. *US Armed Forces Med J* 1953; 4: 31-38.
5. *Epidemiology Bulletin*, Dhahran, Saudi Arabia: Aramco Medical Department, Oct. 1972: 1-2.
6. **Daggy RH.** *Oasis malaria* (Third Conference of the Industrial Council of Tropical Health, Harvard School of Public Health). Industry and Tropical Health III 1957; 3: 49-56.
7. **Daggy RH.** Malaria in oases of eastern Saudi Arabia. *Am J Trop Med Hyg* 1959; 8: 223-291.
8. **Farid MA.** The implications of *Anopheles sergenti* for malaria eradication programmes east of the Mediterranean. *Bull WHO* 1956; 15: 821-827.
9. **Daggy RH.** Malariometric evidence of DDT resistance in *Anopheles stephensi* in cases of Eastern Saudi Arabia. In: *Proceedings of the Sixth International Congress of Tropical Medicine and Malaria.* Lisbon, Portugal, 1958.
10. *Epidemiology Bulletin,* Dhahran, Saudi Arabia: Aramco Medical Department, Nov 1974: 1-3.
11. **Gelpi AP.** Agriculture, malaria and human evolution. A study of genetic polymorphisms in the Saudi oasis population. *Saudi Med J* 1983; 4: 229-234.
12. *Malaria control program in the Kingdom of Saudi Arabia 1983.* Malaria Department, Ministry of Health, Riyadh, 1948: 9-28.
13. **Magzoub M.** *Plasmodium falciparum and Plasmodium vivax* infections in Saudi Arabia, with a note on the distribution of anopheline vectors. *J Trop Med Hyg* 1980; 83: 203-206.
14. *Intercountry malaria meetings of representatives from the Arab States of the Gulf Area.* Official report, Malaria Department, Ministry of Health, Riyadh, Oct 1977: 1-3.
15. *Report on malaria control program in the Kingdom of Saudi Arabia, 1979.* Malaria Department, Ministry of Health, Riyadh, 1980: 1-5.

16. *Malaria control program in the Kingdom of Saudi Arabia, 1983.* Malaria Department, Ministry of Health, Riyadh, 1984: 9-54.

17. **Carson RL.** *Silent spring.* Greenwich Conn Fawcett Publications 1962: pp. 304.

18. Anonymous. *Informal consultation of planning strategy for the prevention of pesticide poisoning.* Geneva: World Health Organization 1986, WHO/VBC/86.926: 28 pp.

19. **Farid MA.** *Malaria in Saudi Arabia.* Malaria Department, Ministry of Health, Riyadh, 1982: 16-19.

SCHISTOSOMIASIS

INTRODUCTION

Schistosomiasis, or bilharziasis, is a helminthic infection of the mesenteric, portal, and pelvic venous systems. The infection has been demonstrated in the mummies of Ancient Egypt and the etiology was known in 1851 by Bilharz who discovered the adult worm in the mesenteric veins of an Egyptian. The life cycle involves man as the primary host and an aquatic snail as the intermediate host. The main pathological effects are the progressive damage to various organs resulting from immunological reactions to the eggs and the parasite deposited in the tissue. Liver cirrhosis and portal hypertension occur in the intestinal form, while obstruction and superimposed infection occur in the urinary form.

Schistosoma mansoni occurs mainly in Africa, the Arabian Peninsula, South America and the Caribbean Islands, while S. haematobium occurs mainly in Africa and the Middle East. Schistosoma japonicum occurs in the Orient, and S. mekongi in Laos, Cambodia and Thailand. About 200 million people in 74 countries are affected; half of them in Africa alone.[1] Despite the extensive knowledge of the life cycle, pathogenesis and methods of prevention, the disease, globally, is not yet under control. The reasons are inefficient management and lack of political commitments and social awareness.

HISTORY

As a medical student in Egypt, I was questioning a patient admitted to the hospital with severe chest pains. After taking down the relevant history I asked him if he had any other complaints. This he denied. I then asked him the classic question for an Egyptian patient, "Do you have blood in your urine?" The answer was "of course I have blood in my urine." This chronic and insidious feature of the disease and the deceptively peaceful coexistence between man and the parasite (at least in the early stages) probably leads to apathy in the patients and the public towards the disease.

Historians have taken little interest in schistosomiasis in the Arabian Peninsula compared to other fatal, disfiguring or painful diseases such as smallpox, cholera, leprosy, plague or malaria. One of the earliest observations of the disease was made by Hatch, an Indian physician in 1887, who noticed *Bilharzia haematobium* infection among pilgrims returning from Makkah.[2] In 1903 Clemow[3] reported that, "there are some reasons to believe that it (schistosomiasis) is common in Arabia." This statement was based on reports from Turkish sanitary officers stationed in Arabia. Later on in 1940, Aramco (Arabian American Oil Company) health officers observed an increasing number of schistosomiasis cases among laborers working in the Eastern Province.

In 1950 Abdul Azim,[4] a WHO consultant, reported that S. *haematobium* and S. *mansoni* were endemic in the fertile areas of Saudi Arabia. He identified the vector snails and envisaged that the extension of irrigation and the oil industry, with the inevitable concentration of population, would intensify the disease. Tarizzo[5] in 1952 scrutinized the records of more than 70,000 Aramco employees and indicated the presumptive place of origin of 893 cases of S. *mansoni* and 51 cases of S. *haematobium*. He identified over 25 localities all over the country with the exception of the Eastern Province where no autochthonous infection was found. In 1956, Tarizzo carried out the first field trial of treatment.[6]

Farouq[7] surveyed selected areas of the country in 1960. He reported a high prevalence of the disease in Al Kharj, Dariya, Taif, Wadi Fatma, Tabuk and Tayma. His conclusion was that bilharziasis in Saudi Arabia is easy to control since the foci of infection are well defined and therefore lend themselves to focal control and even eradication within a relatively short period.

Alio[8] in 1965 carried out an extensive survey on schistosomiasis in Saudi Arabia. His survey allowed a delineation of the endemic areas by finding the vector snails and diagnosing the autochthonous cases.

Sources of infection in Saudi Arabia were classified as natural and man-made foci. The natural foci were further subclassified into permanent foci mainly in the perennial mountain streams and springs, temporary foci usually in the intermittent streams, and transitory foci in the ephemeral flood waters.

Alio[8] estimated the prevalence of the disease among the settled population as up to 90% in Jouf and Sakakah, Ghamid and Zahran Highlands, Bisha oasis, Asir Highland, Tihamat Asir and Najran; 10% in Southern Najd; 5% in Northern Hijaz and Northern Najd and none in the Eastern Province. The total number of individuals presumed to be infected was estimated at 1,024,200 or 17% of the total population. He also believed that this was still a conservative estimate. Alio concluded that the problem of schistosomiasis was quite serious in comparison to many other health problems in Saudi Arabia. For the control of the disease he suggested upgrading environmental sanitation, training of personnel, planned use of molluscicides, and treatment of patients.

In the early 1970s several small scale studies of the disease were conducted. Arfaa[9] and Davis[10] referred to Gizan and Madinah as highly endemic areas of S. haematobium, and Riyadh, Madinah, Makkah and Jouf as endemic foci of S. mansoni. The estimated overall prevalence in the two studies ranged from 2% in Zulfi to 91% in Khoba. They both described the distribution as patchy with rare mixed infection, and thought that eradication was feasible in many parts of the Kingdom.

The studies conducted by Habib et al.,[11] Magzoub and Kasim,[12] Wallace,[13] Gremillon et al.,[14] Cutajar,[15] Ibrahim and Sebai[16] and Hanash et al.[17] were of a clinical nature. They shed light on some features of the pathology, diagnosis and epidemiology of the disease.

Wallace[13] and Cutajar[15] came to some common conclusions; viz: a low prevalence of the disease among females (4-5%), no correlation between urinary schistosomiasis and carcinoma of the uroepithelium; and the relative ease with which the disease can be controlled. On the contrary Hanash et al.[17] reported 30 patients with bilharzial bladder cancer. Cutajar[15] found that schistosomiasis does not appear to be a significant etiological factor in urolithiasis which has a high incidence in Saudi Arabia.

Magzoub and Kasim[12] observed that water bodies do not show any apparent overlap between the different snail vectors of schistosomiasis whereas Arfaa found up to three species of snail (intermediate hosts) together in some areas (personal communication). Germillon *et al.*[14] emphasized the value of quantitative examination of stool specimens for schistosomiasis eggs.

In the 1980s most of the epidemiological data was compiled by Arfaa[18, 19] and Githaiga.[20]

THE PRESENT SITUATION

SNAIL VECTORS

Four species of snail vectors exist in the country. *Biomphlaria arabica*, the intermediate host of *S. mansoni*, is a related species to *Biomphlaria alexandria* which prevails in Egypt, and has its main habitat in Central Arabia and the North and South Western Regions.

The other three species which transmit *S. haematobium* are *Bulinus truncatus* found mainly in the Western Region, *Bulinus reticulatus* found mainly in the Central Region, and *Bulinus bacarri* found mainly in the Central and South Western Regions. The disease distribution follows the snail vector distribution.

THE THEORY OF DISEASE DISSEMINATION

The Arabian Peninsula desert is covered by shifting sands on a high, barren and dry plateau. The rainfall is less than 12.70 cm (5 in) per year, consisting of one monsoon in the winter in the interior of the peninsula and two monsoons in the winter and summer over the southern part of the Sarawat mountains.

Water resources consist of streams, small canals, springs, water holes, dug wells, pools and ponds.

The country could be divided into the following geographic regions: the Red Sea coastal plains, the Sarawat mountains, the central Arabian plateau, the great sand areas (the great Nafud in the north, Rub'al Khali in the south and Dahana desert belt in between), and the Gulf basin.

Saudi Arabia is located between two of the major endemic schistosomiasis areas in the world, the Nile river valley and the Tigris and Euphrates valleys. Evidence indicates that the endemicity of the disease goes back more than 3,000 years in Egypt and over 6,000 years in Iraq, and the type of natural habitats and characteristics of snails suggest the presence of the snails in Saudi Arabia for the same length of time as in the Nile, Tigris and Euphrates valleys.

There are also foci of schistosomiasis in surrounding countries, namely Iraq, Lebanon, Syria, occupied Palestine, Yemen, Ethiopia, Somalia and Sudan. Over time, the disease has crossed the borders of the Arabian Peninsula by means of population movements, pilgrimage and trade.

The main natural habitat of the vector snails appears to be in the Sarawat Mountains where there are various natural water sources such as permanent streams, ponds and springs. The snails disseminate along the major flood routes from the natural water sources in the Sarawat Mountains and fill the wadi beds in the plains. Water often overflows into man-made wells and cisterns and introduces snails to man-made habitats.

At least three important wadis (flood water courses) run through the peninsula towards the East until they are interrupted by the sand belt; Wadi Al Rummah, Wadi Hanifa and Wadi Al Dawasir. They carry the snails to the oases and villages scattered along their courses. Snails are disseminated to other oases and villages through a gradual progression from one suitable water source to another or by means of periodic seasonal floods. The Eastern Province of Saudi Arabia is free from all the snail vectors and the disease, possibly protected by the sand belt separating it from the rest of the country and the high salinity of the soil.

Interestingly, the sand belt in Saudi Arabia delineates the disease distribution. To the West (the African Continent and Western and Central Arabia) schistosomiasis is endemic. To the East of the sand belt, which includes the Eastern Province of Saudi Arabia and the vast majority of the Asian continent, the disease is scarcely found with the exception of Iraq and small foci in Iran and India. In the Far East another species of the parasites and its vector snail appear.

PREVALENCE

In developing countries, data on morbidity and mortality are not always complete. Lack of standardization and inadequate training and supervision of personnel are inherent problems of epidemiological surveys in developing countries.

Statistics on schistosomiasis in Saudi Arabia are not exceptions to the rule. There are 12 schistosomiasis stations located at Riyadh, Jouf, Makkah, Madinah, Taif, Hail, Mahael, Bishah, Abha, Al-Baha, Gizan and Najran. The health personnel in these stations conduct epidemiological surveys, but it must be noted that they vary in their competence, training, motivation and the degree of supervision they receive.

The methods of survey vary from passive case detection (examining patients attending hospitals and health centers) to surveying a whole community or a school. Samples are not always representative and laboratory tests are not necessarily standardized.[20] Nevertheless, the available data still indicate the magnitude of the problem. Table 1 and Fig. 1 show the prevalence of schistosomiasis in various regions in Saudi Arabia as reported by stations in 1983-1984.[19]

Out of 230,802 people examined by all stations, 15,106 were positive for either *S. mansoni or S. haematobium* (an overall prevalence of 6.5%). There are about 2,000,000 people at risk (mostly living in rural areas) and the estimated number of infected people is within the range of 150,000 to 200,000. The disease has a patchy distribution (the prevalence rate within a region ranges from 0 to 80%). The determining factors are the suitability of the habitats for the vector, the abundance of vector snails and the lifestyle of the people.

The disease in general is predominant among the lower age group and affects males more than females. There is a seasonal fluctuation of incidence which follows rainfalls. The infection rate is heavy along the permanent and main streams, and moderate to low in remote areas.

PROBLEMS

As a result of the socioeconomic development and the schistosomiasis control program, a general reduction of the vector snails and the morbidity rate has been noticed especially in the last 5 years (Table 2). An exacerbation of the disease in an area is recorded from time to time as a result of an influx of foreign laborers or a change in the ecosystem. In Taif, where the prevalence rate is 3.8%, the examination of 2277 new expatriates (Egyptians, Sudanese and Yemenis) revealed that 37% were positive.[18]

Table 1. Prevalence of Schistosomiasis as Reported by the Stations.

Station	No. of Persons Examined	Prevalence Rate %		Overall Prevalence*
		S. haematobium	*S. mansoni*	
Al Baha	20,412	—	13.0	13.0
Gizan	30,883	7.0	1.2	8.2
Taif	39,599	0.2	7.7	7.9
Abha	23,013	1.7	4.9	6.6
Madinah	17,591	1.9	3.6	5.5
Bishah	16,766	0.4	8.5	8.9
Najran	8,820	1.6	9.9	11.5
Mahael	5,783	7.6	—	7.6
Hail	4,335	—	14.2	12.2
Riyadh	15,129	—	5.6	5.6
Makkah	25,894	2.5	3.0	5.5
Al Jouf	12,577	1.3	1.6	2.9

Modified from Ref. 19.

*Approximate, since a small percentage has double infection.

Table 2. Changes in Schistosomiasis Infection in Selected Areas in Saudi Arabia: 1974-1984.

	Prevalence Rate %		
	1974	1982	1984
S. haematobium			
Gizan - Ardah	43.5	13.0	6.5
- Khoba	91.0	30.4	13.0
Tayma	58.0	2.0	1.8
S. mansoni			
Al-Hauta	21.0	20.0	2.3
Al-Hareeq	50.0	34.0	3.5

An outstanding example of the possible effect of ecological changes is found in Al Baha area. Three years after Al Sadr Dam was completed in 1981, high infestation with both *B. arabica* and *B. truncatus* was observed both in the lake behind the dam and downstream in the wadi. Eight of the

14 dams completed by 1985 in Al Baha area, became infested with the snail intermediate host (Sebai ZA, personal observation).

Twenty-two projects of dam construction, irrigation schemes and land reclamation are presently proceeding in Saudi Arabia. Unless the impact of the ecological changes is well studied, an expansion of the disease is highly predictable. In the Eastern Province (a schistosomiasis-free area at present) the possibility of introducing the intermediate host exists. This could happen because of the expansion of the irrigation system and the free and fast movements of Bedouins who might carry the vector, for example, in their water skin bags.

The change in the disease pattern following changes in the environment is well documented. A village in the Nile delta was surveyed in 1935 and 1979 for schistosomiasis. During the 44-year period, *S. mansoni* infection increased from 3.2% to 73% and *S. hematobium* infection decreased from 74% to 2.2%. The change has been attributed to a change in the ecosystem after the construction of the Aswan High Dam.[21]

In some communities, adults employed in farming have a high risk of infection. Females in Bedouin communities who carry water to their homes and herd animals in infested wadis are more exposed than men in the same community to the infection.

WHICH WAY FORWARD?

Progress in controlling the disease has already been achieved in the last 20 years. It is, however, the opinion of many researchers (e.g. Farouq,[7] Alio,[8] Davis[10] and Arfaa[9]) that the problem could be completely controlled or even eradicated since the habitats of the vector snails are generally localized. The three bases for further and substantial success are better management, training of personnel, and multifaceted control approach with emphasis on the environmental modification. The collection of reliable data is extremely important in order to improve planning and monitoring.

Research programs are needed in the areas of operational methodology, understanding the lifestyle of the population, developing a vaccine, and even the manipulation of the genetic make-up of the vector snail.

Primary Health Care centers should be upgraded to give maintenance and continuity to schistosomiasis control programs. They should promote health education, active case finding, sanitary engineering, and community participation. By the year 2000 schistosomiasis need not be a problem in Saudi Arabia.

REFERENCES

1. **Mott KE.** Schistosomiasis - new goals. *Magazine WHO Dec.* 1984: 3-4.
2. **Hatch WK.** Bilharzia haematobium. *Lancet* 1887; 1: 875.
3. **Clemow FG.** *The geography of disease.* London: Cambridge University Press, 1903: 570 pp.
4. **Abdel Azim M, Gismann A.** Bilharziasis survey in south-western Asia. *Bull WHO* 1956; 14: 403-456.
5. **Tarizzo ML.** Schistosomiasis in Saudi Arabia. *Vemes. Congres Internationaux de Medecine Tropical et du Paludisme* (Excerpt) 1956.
6. **Tarizzo ML.** Schistosomiasis in Saudi Arabia: treatment with lucanthone hydrochloride (nilodin) and with sodium antimonyl gluconate (triostam). *Am J Trop Med Hyg* 1956; 6: 145-149.
7. **Farooq M.** Report on a visit to Saudi Arabia. *WHO Assignment Report* 1961; EM/BIL/19/SA24: 21 pp.
8. **Alio IS.** *Epidemiology of Schistosomiasis in Saudi Arabia with emphasis on geographic distribution patterns.* Dhahran: Aramco, 1967. 217 pp. Dissertation. NYC, Columbia Univ.
9. **Arfaa F.** Studies on Schistosomiasis in Saudi Arabia. *Am J Trop Med Hyg* 1976; 25 (2): 295-298.
10. **Davis A.** *Schistosomiasis* control in the Kingdom of Saudi Arabia with special reference to chemotherapy. *WHO Assignment Report* 1977.
11. **Habib MA, Morsy TA, El Nayal NA, Shoura MI.** Study of the clinical pattern of bilharziasis in Saudi Arabia. *J Egypt Soc Parasitol* 1977; 7: 163-170.
12. **Magzoub M, Kasim AA.** Schistosomiasis in Saudi Arabia. *Ann Trop Med Parasitol* 1980; 74 (5): 511-513.
13. **Wallace DM.** Urinary *Schistosomiasis* in Saudi Arabia. *Ann R Coll Surg Eng* 1979; 61: 265-270.
14. **Gremillon DH, Geckler RW, Kuntz RE, Marraro RV.** Schistosomiasis in Saudi Arabian recruits, a morbidity study based on quantitative egg excretion. *Am J Trop Med Hyg* 1978; 27 (5): 924-927.
15. **Cutajar CL.** Urinary Schistosomiasis in the Asir district of Saudi Arabia. In: Mahjoub ES ed. *Proceedings of the 5th Saudi Medical*

Meeting Riyadh: College of Medicine, University of Riyadh, 1981: 543-552.

16. **Ibrahim AM, Sebai ZA,** Analytic study of patients attending the bilharzia clinic in Riyadh, Saudi Arabia. SMJ 1978; 16: 14-12.

17. **Hanash KA, Bissada NK, Abla A, Esmail D, Dowling A.** Predictive values of excretory urography, ultrasonography, computerized tomography, and liver and bone scan in the staging of bilharzial bladder cancer in Saudi Arabia. *Cancer* 1984; 54: 172-176.

18. **Arfaa F.** Schistosomiasis control in the Kingdom of Saudi Arabia. WHO *Assignment Report* 1984; EM/SCHIS/89-SAA/MPD/002.

19. **Arfaa F.** Schistosomiasis control programme in the Kingdom of Saudi Arabia. WHO *Assignment Report 1984;* EM/SCHIS/SAA/MPD/002.

20. **Githaiga HK.** *Fact finding visits to bilharzia centers in the Kingdom of Saudi Arabia.* Report to the Ministry of Health Department of Preventive Medicine - Bilharziasis Section 1984.

21. **Abdel-Wahab MF.** Changing pattern of Schistosomiasis in Egypt 1935-79. *Lancet* 1979; 4: 242-4.

Figure 1. The overall prevalence of intestinal and urinary Schistosomiasis in various parts of Saudi Arabia - 1984.

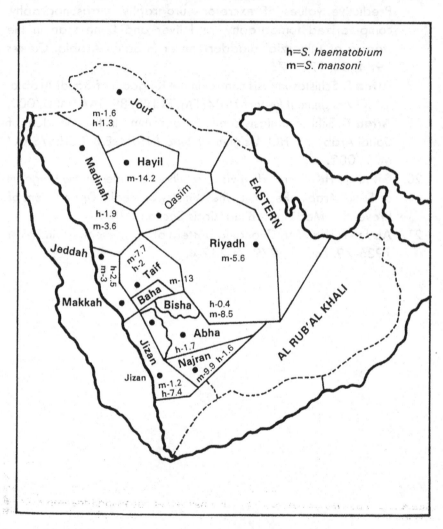

Source: 19 modified.

TUBERCULOSIS

INTRODUCTION

Tuberculosis is an ancient disease; its pathological changes have been found in the skeletons of Neolithic man. The disease is caused by *Mycobacterium tuberculosis* and the principal source of infection is from persons with active pulmonary tuberculosis. The lungs are the most common site of primary infection, but extrapulmonary tuberculosis, especially in the alimentary tract, may occur either primarily or secondary to pulmonary disease. The clinical manifestations of the disease are the result of the continuing battle between the invading mycobacterium and the host's defense mechanism. Childhood infection is now thought not to confer lifetime protection from exogenous reinfection, as was previously believed.[1]

Tuberculosis, although declining in importance as a problem in industrialized countries, still constitutes a major problem in the developing world. According to the World Health Organization (WHO),[2] the annual incidence rate varies widely from 0.03% in industrialized countries to 1.5% in some developing countries. Each year 3.5 million people contract the disease and about 0.5 million die. The mortality rate varies from 75 per 100,000 in the Philippines to 0.9 per 100,000 in Australia.

The morbidity and mortality rate from tuberculosis declined in the Western hemisphere well before the introduction of anti-tuberculosis chemotherapy. This decline has been attributed to socioeconomic development and improvements in housing, nutrition and working conditions. Treatment on an out-patient basis can be very effective if combined with preventive measures, including better housing and nutrition, early case finding, immunization of infants, chemoprophylaxis of contacts and the improvement of the self-reliance of the people.

Although gastrointestinal tuberculosis has become rare in the Western world, it still imposes a problem in developing countries. The primary lesion is caused by bovine mycobacterium bacilli ingested as a result of consuming unpasteurized milk from household goats and cows. Secondary infection resulting from a tuberculous focus elsewhere in the body is globally declining as a result of effective anti-tuberculous treatment.[3]

PREVALENCE

The epidemiological data on tuberculosis in Saudi Arabia are quite meagre. Our present knowledge is derived from limited studies carried out in small communities, hospitals or schools. In the absence of a National sample survey and a reliable notification system these studies remain the source of our information.

The observations made by a WHO consultant on the health situation in Saudi Arabia in 1949 are of historical interest.[4] In the country at that time there were only 111 physicians (over 14,000 in 1986) and 1,000 beds (over 31,000 in 1986). Tuberculosis, trachoma and venereal disease (most likely bejel) were stated to be the three main health problems in Saudi Arabia but no statistics were given. There were no special hospital beds for tuberculosis patients and X-ray equipment was available only in Makkah, Riyadh and Dhahran.

Few studies based on tuberculin skin tests have been conducted in local communities in order to explore the rate of infection. In a study conducted in 1967 in the rural community of Turaba, Western Saudi Arabia,[5] the tine tuberculin test was applied to 387 persons. The frequency of positive reactions (>2mm in duration) ranged from 12% among pre-school children to 70% among adults.

In a study of the rural community of Barza, Western Saudi Arabia,[6] positive reactions to the tuberculin test ranged from 1.9% among children 6-9 years of age, to 32% among persons above 15 years of age.

At a military school in Tabuk 125 first year students were studied.[7] Less than 10% were positive to the Mantoux test, mostly associated with

Bacillus Calmette-Guerin (BCG) vaccination. Another survey of tuberculin sensitivity was conducted among 6 to 19-year-old boys at the military schools in Riyadh.[8] Of 893 boys tested, 433 (49%) were positive to the tine test. Over 80% of the positives had evidence of previous BCG vaccination. No active cases of tuberculosis were detected.

In Turaba and Barza, both rural communities where BCG vaccination was not commonly practiced, a high percentage of the people contracted the infection. Nevertheless one has to consider infection with non-specific mycobacteria as a possible cause of the positive reactions. In the Riyadh and Tabuk studies, the BCG vaccination concealed the evidence of natural infection.

In 1971 a study of tuberculosis in the schools of Riyadh revealed a 1.5%-2.5% prevalence rate of suspicious radiological shadows.[9] If this figure were to be generalized, there would be about 150,000 radiologically active tuberculosis in the Kingdom, 25-33% of which are likely to be bacteriologically positive. The author concluded that tuberculosis is a leading cause of morbidity and a major public health problem in Saudi Arabia. However, it must be borne in mind that the whole socioeconomic status of the country is very different now (1986), and thus along with other considerations the previous extrapolation seems to be out of place.

There are indications that the prevalence of the disease has decreased in recent years. From the reports of the Arabian American Oil Company (Aramco), in the Eastern Province[10] the rate of active pulmonary tuberculosis cases decreased from 230 per 100,000 in 1957 to 40 per 100,000 in 1976. According to the Ministry of Health Annual Report (1979)[11] the incidence of tuberculosis in Saudi Arabia has declined from 1299 per 100,000 in 1970 to 166 per 100,000 in 1979. This figure should be considered as an estimate since it is based on reports from tuberculosis centers rather than an actual survey.

In 1981-1982, a retrospective study was conducted on 47 tuberculous Saudi patients (25 males, 22 females) attending the Department of Primary Care, Riyadh Military Hospital.[12] The distribution of the lesions was pulmonary: 57%; nodal: 19%; bone and spine: 11%; miliary: 4% and peritoneal: 9%. Pulmonary tuberculosis was more common among males while the non-pulmonary form was more common among females (p<.0.01). No explanation for this difference was given. Only 16 of the 47 cases (34%) were clinically suspected of having tuberculosis, an indication of the need for an active detection programme. The fact that

14 patients (30%) had a history of previously treated disease indicated a poor compliance of patients to treatment.

In 1982, a trial was made to assess the magnitude of the tuberculosis problem in the Arab countries. The area was divided into three categories; Saudi Arabia, Yemen, Oman, Sudan and Somalia were among the highest incidence group. The incidence of active cases was estimated at 1% per year.[13] Another study at the same time referred to tuberculosis as the most important infectious disease in Saudi Arabia.[14]

Extrapulmonary tuberculosis has been the subject of some studies. The studies were hospital-based, hence the focus was clinical rather than epidemiological. Of the total 10,719 cases of tuberculosis seen at all tuberculosis centers in the Kingdom during the period 1975-1979, 78% were pulmonary tuberculosis and 22% were non-pulmonary tuberculosis.[11]

Over a 3-year period (1978-1980) 845 cases of tuberculosis were diagnosed at King Abdul Aziz University Hospital in Jeddah.[15] Of the total, 125 (15%) had extrapulmonary tuberculosis. The distribution of the lesions was nodal: 68; abdominal: 20; urogenital: 16; renal: 4; bones and joints: 12 and miscellaneous: 5. The age range was 5 to 75 years (average 22 years); male to female ratio 3 to 1, and Saudi to non-Saudi 4 to 1. Most of the Saudis came from rural areas.

In contrast to the above mentioned findings, of the 82 cases of all types of tuberculosis admitted to King Khalid University Hospital, Riyadh during the year 1983, only 21% were pulmonary and 79% were non-pulmonary tuberculosis (Abdullah AK, unpublished observations). Apparently the results from the two university hospitals in Jeddah and Riyadh do not reflect the general situation in the Kingdom.

A study in Makkah and Jeddah hospitals over a 12-year period (1969-1980) revealed 18 cases with gastrointestinal tuberculosis.[16] The consumption of unpasteurized or boiled milk is still practiced among the rural population of Saudi Arabia with the belief that it is more natural and healthy.

Tuberculosis involvement of the spine, although relatively uncommon, is often one of the most serious and dangerous manifestations of the disease. Sixty-two patients with tuberculosis of the spine were reported from King Faisal Specialist Hospital over a 3-year period from 1978-1980.[17] There were 38 males and 24 females with an average age of 39 years. The distribution of the lesions was thoracic: 50%; lumbar: 25%; cervical: 13% and in the thoracolumbar junction: 8%. Thirty-six patients

(58%) presented with tetraparesis or paraparesis, an indication of late diagnosis.

Only one case of Takayasus disease (Type III) affecting an Arab male was reported.[18] The patient had previously suffered from tuberculosis which is thought to be a possible etiological basis for this form of arteritis affecting major vessels.

CONTROL

In 1949, tuberculosis was considered one of the three main health problems in the country.[4] At that time the health resources were at a minimum and there was no organized health care for the tuberculous patients. The recommendations were: the need for data collection, mass screening, BCG vaccination, the establishment of clinics, and the training of personnel.

In 1960, the Ministry of Health developed a joint project with the World Health Organization to carry out a control program. By the early 1970s some progress had been made on the curative side, but preventive measures were lagging behind.[19]

In 1984, a WHO consultant, reported the following observations:[20]

1. There is no organized program for control of tuberculosis in the Kingdom.
2. The services are mainly hospital oriented.
3. The general hospitals and primary health care centers are not involved in systematic case finding; the case finding activity stands at about 20% of what should be expected.
4. In Gizan, only 27% of children in the 0-4 years age group underwent BCG vaccination.
5. In Gizan, only 30% of the patients completed their treatment.

By 1985, a magnificent expansion of the health care system was achieved including more than 1,090 hospital beds and 11 health centers assigned for tuberculosis, all equipped with modern facilities. Nevertheless, preventive and promotive aspects were still lagging behind.

However, there are signs of progress, mainly through a growing interest among the authorities to improve control measures and integrate them in the primary health care system.

WHICH WAY FORWARD?

A national tuberculosis control program is required to overcome such a major health problem. To reduce morbidity and mortality due to the disease, accurate data on the magnitude and distribution of the problem should be obtained. A national sampling survey and reliable reporting system are vital. Health personnel in various disciplines (both epidemiological and clinical) need to be trained to collect, analyze and disseminate data, administer curative and preventive programs, and follow up and evaluate progress.

The integration of the control program (curative, preventive and promotive) in a well-developed primary health care system is the answer to many problems. Such a system can promote active case finding, BCG vaccination for infants and preventative treatment for contacts. The treatment of 90% of sputum positive cases can be achieved effectively on an out-patient basis. Self-reliance of citizens should be encouraged so that the community shares the responsibility for all aspects of care.

Expatriate laborers and pilgrims, many of whom come from underdeveloped countries, need special attention in terms of screening before entering the country, periodical check-ups, and provision of proper environment in work and at home. Nomadic Bedouins require mobile clinics or health posts connected to the primary health care system. The control of bovine tuberculosis requires a close examination of livestock and improvement of veterinary medicine.

The use of Islamic values, which emphasize cleanliness and personal hygiene, could be very effective in health education programs. Islam recognizes cleanliness as a pillar of faith. For example the Prophet Mohammad 'peace be upon Him', preached His followers to cover the nose and the mouth while sneezing or coughing. It has been recently documented that covering the nose or mouth when sneezing or coughing dramatically reduces the possibility of a droplet infection.[21]

Finally, cooperation between the Gulf countries in applying control measures has to be strengthened in order to fight against a disease which easily crosses territorial borders.

REFERENCES

1. **Davidson PT.** Tuberculosis, new views of an old disease. *New Engl J Med* 1985; 312: 1514-1515.

2. Anonymous. *Sixth report on the world health situation 1973-1977* Part I: global analysis. (Arabic) Geneva: World Health Organization 1982: 112-114.

3. **Abrams JS, Holden WD.** Tuberculosis of the gastrointestinal tract. *Arch Surg* 1964; 89: 282-293.

4. **Papanikalaou B.** *The tuberculosis control program in Saudi Arabia.* WHO/TBC/10; 1949: 20-23.

5. **Sebai ZA.** *The health of the family in changing Arabia.* Jeddah: Tihama Publications, 1983: 93-95.

6. **Hammam HM, Kamel LM and Hidayat NM.** A health profile of a rural community in the Western Zone of Saudi Arabia. In: *Proceedings of the 4th Saudi Medical Conference.* Dammam: King Faisal University, 1980: 35-49.

7. **Grimes J, Sparrow JY, Woodbine A.** Program of health education and health screening in schools. *Saudi Child* 1980; 1: 22-28.

8. **Rowlands DF.** Tuberculosis sensitivity in a Saudi military school population. *Saudi Med J* 1984; 5: 183-189.

9. **Gultekin MS.** Tuberculosis control. *WHO Assignment Report* 1971, EM/TB/119. 25 pp.

10. **Aramco Medical Department.** Active pulmonary tuberculosis cases reported by Aramco health facilities, 1956-1976. *Epidemiology Bull* 1976: 1-3.

11. The Ministry of Health, Kingdom of Saudi Arabia. *Ann Rep* 1399H. (1979): 199-358.

12. **Shanks NJ, Khalifa I, Al Kalai D.** Tuberculosis in Saudi Arabia. *Saudi Med J* 1983; 4: 151-156.

13. **Rifai E.** *Tuberculosis in Arab countries.* Al Majallah Al Tibbiah Al Saudia (Arabic) 1982; 1: 86.

14. **Froude JRL, Kingston M.** Extra pulmonary tuberculosis in Saudi Arabia: a review of 162 cases. *King Faisal Specialist Hospital Med J* 1982; 2: 85-95.

15. **Salam KM, Bedeiwy AF, Saad A, Merdad.** In: *Proceedings of the 6th Saudi Medical Conference,* Jeddah: King Abdul Aziz University, 1981.

16. **Wazna MF.** Gastrointestinal tuberculosis. *King Abdul Aziz Med J* 1981; 1: 16-73.

17. **Lifeso RC.** Preliminary study of tuberculosis of the spine. *King Faisal Specialist Hospital Med J* 1982; 2: 3-13.

18. **Tongia RK, Fonseca V, Al-Nozha M, Fawzy ME.** Takayasu's disease in an Arab male: relationship with tuberculosis. *Saudi Med J* 1985; 6: 113-118.

19. **Gallen CS.** Assignment report, tuberculosis control, Saudi Arabia. WHO Regional Office for the Eastern Mediterranean, *Saudi Arabia* 1201 (Ex 0013) 1972; 1-8.

20. **Aneja KS.** Tuberculosis in Saudi Arabia: WHO *Assignment Rep* EM/TB/164-SAA/ESD/001. 1984: 3-4.

21. **Comstock GW.** Tuberculosis. In: Last JM (ed.) *Maxcy-Rosenau Public Health and Preventive Medicine.* 11th ed. New York: Appleton-Century-Crofts, 1980: 205-220.

VIRAL HEPATITIS (TYPE B)

There are two distinct types of viral hepatitis, **hepatitis A** (previously known as infectious hepatitis) and **hepatitis** B (previously known as serum hepatitis). Other viruses known to be hepatotrophic are non-A and non-B, cytomegalo, Epstein-Barr, herpes simplex and yellow fever viruses. In this chapter we will discuss the most pathogenic type, hepatitis B virus (HBV).

Hepatitis B constitutes a major health problem throughout the world, particularly in the developing world including the Middle Eastern countries. It is estimated that there are about 200 million carriers of HBV throughout the world or approximately 5% of the Earth's population. The prevalence rate ranges from 0.1% in North America to 20% or more in areas of Africa and Asia.

In countries where HBV is uncommon, infection rarely occurs before adulthood, while in countries of high HBV frequency, infection occurs most often in early childhood. Within each country or region considerable differences in prevalence may exist between different ethnic and socioeconomic groups. Hepatitis B Virus (HBV) was originally called the Dane particle (HBV). It possesses three separate antigens.

1.   Hepatitis B surface antigen (ABsAg) (formerly Australia antigen) found on the surface of the virus. Its presence in serum indicates active infection and implies infectivity of the blood. Several

subtypes of HBsAg exist (adr, ayr, adw, ayw) that are of epidemiologic interest but have little clinical significance.

2. Hepatitis B core antigen (HBcAg) is associated with the viral inner core. It can be found in infected liver cells but is not detectable in serum except by special techniques which describe the Dane particle.

3. The antigen HBeAg is closely associated with virus B, but its exact origin is still unknown. It is found only in HBsAg-positive serum and its presence may be associated with greater infectivity of the blood and a strong probability of chronic liver disease.

Hepatitis may be diagnosed by the specific finding of HBsAg in serum in the acute phase of illness or in the carrier state. The presence of anti-HBs or anti-HBc in serum is indicative of antecedent infection.

Methods of the virus transmission include blood transfusion, parenteral drugs, sexual contact especially among promiscuous heterosexuals and male homosexuals, tattooing and ear-piercing, hemodialysis and vertical transmission from an infected mother to her baby. The incubation period is 2—6 weeks. Most affected individuals have asymptomatic infection. For the symptomatic patients the pre-icteric phase is manifested by profound anorexia, nausea, vomiting and vague epigastric discomfort.

Three general patterns of serologic and clinical responses to infection are found: (a) asymptomatic infection, (b) acute hepatitis with a 95% recovery within 6 months and (c) development of chronic carrier state in 5% of the patients. The majority of the chronic carriers are healthy but spread the disease whereas a small fraction may develop complications including liver cirrhosis, primary liver cell carcinoma or immune-complex diseases such as glomerulonephritis and polyarthritis nodosa.

Since 1968 when the association was made between the Australia antigen, now known as hepatitis B surface antigen (HBsAg), and serum hepatitis, there has been considerable advance in knowledge of the nature of the disease. A surface antigen vaccine has recently been developed but its cost is very high.

During the last 5 years viral hepatitis in Saudi Arabia has become a subject of interest to several researchers. However, all the studies have been conducted on selected populations and localities. More comprehensive studies are still needed for better understanding of the etiology, transmission, prevalence and methods of control of the disease.

Table 1 shows the results of studies published in the period between 1980-1985 on the prevalence of the disease in Saudi Arabia.

Jamjoom and Higham (1980)[1] studied antigenemia in two groups of patients in King Abdul-Aziz Hospital in Riyadh. The first group of 233 patients with hepatic abnormalities showed an HBsAg prevalence of 21.9%, and the second group of 424 general patients, 4.5%. The authors concluded that a) viral hepatitis B should be one of the primary considerations in the diagnosis of liver disease in Saudi Arabia, and b) HBsAg occurs in a significantly higher percentage in the serum of patients with symptoms of liver diseases than the other group.

Moaz et al. (1982)[2] examined the sera of 7,894 patients in the Riyadh Al-Kharj Military Hospitals. Of these, 578 (7.3%) were positive for HBsAg (11.9% among males and 5.8% among females). The prevalence increased by age starting at 2.1% in the age group of 0-5 years and reached its peak of 10.6% in the age group of 56-65 years.

Talukder et al. (1982)[3] examined the sera of 3,588 healthy men in the Eastern Province for the presence of HBsAg. The results were positive for 341 (8.8%). Table 2 shows the distribution of his findings according to age groups.

Shafi (1983)[4] compared the prevalence of HBsAg and anti-HBs in two groups, 2,845 Saudi patients attending the National Guard King Khalid Hospital in Jeddah and 639 expatriate hospital staff and their dependents. Out of 2,845

Table 1. Studies Conducted on the Prevalence of HBsAg in Saudi Arabia (1980-1985).

First Author	Ref.	Place	Population Studied	No. Persons	% Positive
Jamjoom	1	Riyadh	Hepatic patients	233	21.4
			General patients	424	4.5
Basalamah	6	Jeddah	Pregnant women	5,000	2.8
Shobokshi	17	Jeddah	Blood donors	850	10.2
Talukder	3	E. Province	General public	3,588	8.8
Shafi	4	Jeddah	General patients	2,845	7.4
Moaz	2	Riyadh	General patients	7,894	7.3
Fathalla	7	E. Province	Selected Groups	24,690	9.8
Fathalla	7	E. Province	(Saudis)	4,712	11.9

Saudi patients, 210 (7.4%) were positive for HBsAg (9.9% of the males and 5.2% of the females). Their age distribution is not different from the findings by Talukder,[3] i.e. low among young and old and highest among the 40-49 years age group. Of 398 HBsAg-negative patients tested, anti-HBc was found in 207 (52%).

Of the 639 expatriate members of the hospital staff and their dependents tested, HBsAg was detected in 1.4% (0.3% among Europeans and 2.7 among Filipinos, Indians and Middle Easterners). The antibody to the HBsAg (anti-HBs) was present in 8.8% of this population.

The author concluded that 59.4% of the Saudi group had experienced HBV infection, 7.4% had HBsAg and 52% carried anti-HBc.

Table 2. Distribution of Carriers of HBsAg Among Male Saudi Arabians by Age.

Age Range (Years)	No. of Patients	No. Positive	(%)
10-15	17	0	
16-25	2,549	218	(8.6)
26-35	767	91	(11.9)
36-45	206	28	(13.6)
46-55	41	4	(9.8)
56-65	6	0	
66	2	0	
Total	**3,588**	**341**	**(8.8)**

From: Ref. 3.

(1953-1962). A high mortality rate was observed among women in general (31% versus 4.5% among men) but an alarmingly high mortality (46.3%) occurred among pregnant women. The author stated that "one disease which appeared especially threatening to Saudis was infectious hepatitis. The mortality from this disease was unexpectedly high among hospitalized males, higher still among adolescent and adult females and alarmingly high among pregnant females." The author compared his findings with those reported from other areas of the Middle East and North Africa, and suggested that Semitic populations may be at considerable risk from fatal hepatitis during pregnancy. It remains a matter for speculation whether this difference reflects an ethnic variation in response to the disease, a geographical difference in the virulence of the virus, or even an expression of subtle nutritional deficiency among women in the Semitic populations.

Gelpi (1979)[12] continued his work with a prospective study (1963-1975) on pregnancy complicated by hepatitis. The investigation of 74 women revealed a striking reduction in mortality compared to his earlier study.[11] However, the risk of fatal hepatitis among pregnant women compared to non-pregnant women remained virtually unchanged.

Although in the literature[13, 14] malnutrition is considered to play an important role in determining the outcome of hepatitis, Gelpi challenged this concept. In his view malnutrition does not explain the increased mortality risk in relation to pregnancy. Also the socioeconomic development which Saudi Arabia experienced in the 1970s, in his opinion, does not completely explain the change in mortality and he concludes "Pregnancy itself seems to be an important determinant of severity and the risk of death with viral hepatitis".

Mallia (1981)[15] followed 48 patients with acute hepatitis in Tabuk Hospital. Out of 15 pregnant women, nine developed fulminating hepatitis resulting in two deaths. The author suggested that pregnant patients having viral hepatitis are at a greater risk of developing fulminating hepatitis in the late stages of pregnancy, but that malnutrition is not a contributing factor to fulminating hepatitis.

Hilton (1980)[16] was interested in the relation between hepatitis B virus and the development of renal diseases. He studied 25 Saudi patients who had end-stage renal disease. Seventeen (68%) were either currently positive for HBsAg or more commonly had evidence of past exposure to hepatitis B. This is significantly higher than his findings among a control group of 32 healthy Saudis (31% positive). Hilton suggested that hepatitis B virus may be an important factor in the development of renal disease in Saudi Arabia. However, the sample size was too small to support such a hypothesis.

DISCUSSION

Most of the studies on hepatitis in Saudi Arabia have been published in the period between 1980-1985, an indication of a recent genuine interest in the problem. Most of these studies have been either published in the *Saudi Medical Journal* or presented in the Annual Saudi Medical Meetings; five of them were carried out by Saudis as main researchers. All are indicative of progressive interest in research. The studies share common limitations, namely small sample sizes, and selected populations. They raise some questions rather than provide answers; in itself a healthy sign as a start. A striking feature is the apparent variability in the prevalence rates of HBsAg among some of the studies. For example, Basalamah et al.[6] and Talukder et al.[3] both used the same technique in studying the prevalence of HBsAg (Reverse Passive Haemagglutination Assay), nevertheless their results were quite different, being 2.8% and 8.8% respectively.

The transmission of infection from HBV carrier mothers to their infants in the perinatal period has been documented as an important mechanism of transmission (vertical transmission). The risk of such perinatal infection may reach 40% in some countries.[5]

Basalamah et al. (1984)[6] tried to find the hepatitis B prevailing sub-type and to investigate the mode of transmission from carrier mothers to their newborn infants.

Table 3. Prevalence of HBsAg in Different Nationalities in the Eastern Province.

Nationality	No. Tested	No. Positive for HBsAg	(%)
Saudi	4,712	560	(11.9)
Yemeni	2,166	298	(13.8)
South Eastern Asia	5,396	674	(12.5)
India Subcontinent	5,928	509	(8.6)
Middle East	2,698	229	(8.5)
West European and USA	1,330	7	(0.5)
Not Known	2,460	141	(5.7)
Total	**24,690**	**2,418**	**(9.8)**

From: Ref. 7.

Of 5,000 Saudi women surveyed antenatally in King Abdulaziz Hospital in Jeddah for HBsAg, 140 (2.8%) were positive. Hepatitis B sub-type ayw was found more often than sub-type adw.

The follow-up of 50 persistent carriers and their newborn infants over a period of two years did not reveal any evidence of materno-fetal transmission either vertically, perinatally or postnatally. The 50 women were tested for HBeAg and anti-HBe antibody. Six (12%) were found to be positive for HBeAg and 42 (92%) for the anti-HBe antibody. The mothers shown to be carrying HBeAg during pregnancy did not apparently transmit the virus to their newborn infants.

Basalamah *et al.*[6] concluded that "materno-foetal transmission of hepatitis B virus *in utero* or during the perinatal period does not seem to be important in maintaining the carrier state in Saudi Arabia, horizontal rather than vertical being the main route of transmission of the virus in this country". The study shed some light on the problem, although the sample size was too small to provide a final conclusion on materno-fetal transmission or the prevailing sub-type.

The most recent and extensive study was conducted by Fathalla *et al.* (1985)[7] in the Eastern Province. A total number of 24,690 persons (blood donors, food handlers, pregnant women and children) of different nationalities were examined; 9.6% were positive for HBsAg. Table 3 shows the distribution of results according to nationality. Out of 4,712 Saudis, 560 (11.9%) were positive. The prevalence rates within the nationality groups seem to reflect the prevalence rates seen in their countries of origin.[8] The authors suggested that blood donors and food handlers may act as important reservoirs of HBV. However, the difference between the prevalence among expatriates in this study and the study of Shafi[4] is striking. Fathalla[7] came to the same conclusion as Basalamah that vertical transmission may be of less importance than horizontal transmission.

The association between primary hepatocellular carcinoma and liver cirrhosis and hepatitis B infection is already documented in the literature.[9] From the records of the Department of Medicine of the Riyadh Armed Forces Hospital,[10] liver cirrhosis and hepatic cell carcinoma are the most common causes of death among patients under the age of 60. One-third of the chronic liver diseases present at the hospital are associated with hepatitis B infections.

Researchers have been interested in the risk of fatal hepatitis during pregnancy. Gelpi (1977)[11] conducted a retrospective study of mortality from viral hepatitis on a group of 764 Saudi Arabian patients admitted to Aramco (Arabian American Oil Company) Hospital, Dhahran, over a 10-year period

The studies conducted by Moaz *et al.*,[2] Shobokshi and Serebour,[17] and Talukder *et al.*,[3] Shafi and Mounsey[4] and Fathalla *et al.*[7] covered over 40,000 Saudi individuals examined in different regions in the country and gave a HBsAg carrier rate between 2.8% and 11.9%. An overall prevalence rate of 8% (the mode) might be a realistic figure as a basis for further investigation and planning purposes.

RECOMMENDATION

Since the epidemiology and mode of transmission of viral hepatitis is not fully understood, manipulation of the environment or the lifestyle cannot provide control with certainty. Treatment is out of question at present and passive immunity (HBIg) is expensive and gives temporary protection. Active immunization is potentially the most effective means of control. Its efficacy rate is almost 100% and it is safe.[18, 19] A committee composed of representatives of the US Center for Disease Control, the US Food and Drug Administration and the US National Institute of Health, reported that hepatitis B vaccine carried minimal immediate side-effects and no long-term reaction.[20] However it is expensive; a full course of three injections costs more than SR 300.

Several researchers[4, 7, 21, 22, 23, 24] called for the use of the vaccine to prevent such an overwhelming disease in Saudi Arabia. The general agreement is that until the time when vaccines become available for all the public, selected groups should be given priority for vaccination. These include:

1. Combined passive-active immunization for newborns of mothers known to be HBsAg chronic carriers or mothers who developed hepatitis in the last trimester or within three months of delivery.
2. Active immunization may be given after screening to the Hepatitis B sero-negatives including:
    a. Mothers attending hospitals, health centers and well-baby clinics.
    b. Household contacts of acute hepatitis cases or HBsAg carriers.
    c. Multiple transfused patients, patients with hemophilia and those on hemodialysis.
    d. Health care personnel who come into contact with potentially infectious patients or their specimens.

At the same time, research work should continue to investigate the magnitude of the problem, and identify those susceptible and those who are at special risk. At present researchers are exploring genetic engineering and synthetic processes to produce a more economic vaccine.[25]

CONCLUSION

It seems that about 60% of the Saudi population have experienced infection with hepatitis B virus; approximately 8% of these are carriers and 52% are healthy individuals showing antibodies in their blood. Susceptibility to the infection increases with age, reaching its peak at 50 years, and is higher among males than females. More comprehensive research is needed for a better understanding of the disease; its etiology, mode of transmission, pathogenesis, prevalence, distribution, and control.

The Southern parts of the country do not seem to have been covered by these studies, which have been conducted mainly in the Eastern and Western Regions. Very few studies are from the Central Region and the North. This geographic distribution of published results should be taken in consideration in future studies.

Considering the high prevalence of the disease and its association with liver cirrhosis and hepatic cell carcinoma, immediate action is required. The launching of a well-directed vaccination program seems to be, at present, the most effective method of control.

REFERENCES

1. **Jamjoom GA, Higham R.** Prevalence of viral hepatitis type B surface antigen (HBsAg) in patients with liver disease and in the general patient population at King Abdulaziz Hospital, Riyadh. In: Mahgoub E, ed. *Proceedings of the 5th Saudi Medical Meeting.* Riyadh: College of Medicine, University of Riyadh, 1980; 331-339.

2. **Moas A, Admaway AMO, Talukder MAS, Gilmore R.** Prevalence of hepatitis in the patient population of Riyadh Al-Kharj Hospitals Programme. In: *Proceedings of the 7th Saudi Medical Meeting.* Dammam: King Faisal University, 1982: 252-255.

3. **Talukder MAS, Gilmore R, Bacchus RA.** Prevalence of hepatitis B surface antigen among male Saudi Arabians. *J Infect Dis* 1982; 146: 446.

4. **Shafi MS, Mounsey G.** Prevalence of hepatitis B virus infection: experience at the National Guard King Khalid Hospital, Jeddah. In: Academic Committee ed *Abstracts of the 8th Saudi Medical Conference,* Riyadh: Saudi National Guard Medical Services Department 1983: 245.

5. **Maynard JE.** Hepatitis. In: Last JM ed. *Maxcy-Rosenau. Public Health and Preventive Medicine* 11th ed. New York: Appleton-Century-Crofts, 1980: 159-165.

6. **Basalamah AH, Serebour F, Kazim E.** Materno-Foetal transmission of hepatitis B in Saudi Arabia. *J Infect* 1984; 8: 200-204.

7. **Fathalla SE, Namnyak SS, Al-Jama AA** *et al.* The prevalence of hepatitis B surface antigen in healthy subjects residing in the Eastern Province of Saudi Arabia. *Saudi Med J* 1985; 6: 236-241.

8. **Sobeslavsky O.** Prevalence of markers of hepatitis B virus infection in various countries: A WHO collaborative study. *Bull Wld Hlth Org* 1980; 58: 621-623.

9. **Beasley RP, Hwang LY, Lin CC, Chien CS.** Hepatocellular carcinoma and hepatitis B virus: A Prospective Study of 22,707 Men in Taiwan. *Lancet* 1981; 1129-33.

10. **Peters RL.** Viral hepatitis: A Pathologic Spectrum. *Am J Med Sci 1975; 270:17-31.*

11. **Gelpi AP.** Fatal hepatitis in Saudi Arabian women. *Am J Gastrol* 1970; 53: 41-61.

12. **Gelpi AP.** Viral hepatitis complicating pregnancy: mortality trends in Saudi Arabia. *Int J Gyn Obs* 1979; 17: 73-77.

13. **Bhalerao VR, Desi VP, Pai DN.** Viral hepatitis in pregnancy. *Ind J Publ Hlth* 1974; 18: 165-70.

14. **Borha F. Haghighi P, Kekmat K, Rezaizadeh K.** Viral hepatitis during pregnancy: severity and effect on gestation. *Gastroenterology* 1973; 64: 304-312.

15. **Mallia C.** Hepatitis in pregnancy. *Br Med J* 1981; 283: 1546.

16. **Hilton PJ, Michael J, Wing AJ, Jones NF, Banatvala JE.** Hepatitis B virus and end-stage renal disease. *New Engl J Med* 1980; 303: 225-626.

17. **Shobokshi O, Serebour F.** Hepatitis B: problem in Saudi Arabia. In: Szmuness W. *et al.* eds. *Viral Hepatitis.* 1981 International Symposium. The Franklin Institute Press (Abstract) 673.

18. **Szmuness W.** Hepatitis B vaccine: demonstration of efficacy in a controlled clinical trial in a high risk population in the United States. *New Engl J Med* 1980; 303 (15): 833-841.

19. **Szmuness W, Stevens CE, Zang EA, Harley EJ, Kellner A.** A controlled clinical trial of the efficacy of the hepatitis B vaccine (Heptavax B): a final report. *Hepatology* 1981; 1: 377-385.

20. Hepatitis B virus vaccine safety: Report of an Interagency Group. *Morbid Mortal Wkly Rep* 1982; 31: 465.

21. **Abdurrahman MB.** Hepatitis B infection and immunization: A Review. *Saudi Med J* 1984; 5: 369-376.

22. **Little PJ.** Hepatitis B vaccination. *Saudi Med J* 1983; 4: 1-4.

23. **Larkworthy W.** Hepatitis B vaccination. *The King Faisal Specialist Hosp Med J* 1983; 3: 85-86.

24. **Haque K.** Hepatitis B vaccination. *Saudi Med J* 1983; 4: 275-276.

25. **Zuckerman AJ.** Priorities for immunization against hepatitis B. *Br Med J* 1982; 284: 686-688.

TRACHOMA

INTRODUCTION

Trachoma affects 15% of the world population and is a leading cause of preventable blindness. The causative agent is *Chlamydia trachomatis* which also causes, with different serotypes, genital tract infection in the Western world.

The disease is defined as a specific communicable keratoconjunctivitis, usually of chronic evolution or even lifetime duration if not treated. It is characterized by the formation of follicles, papillary hyperplasia and pannus, and typically leads to scar formation. Trachoma can cause chronic inflamation of the mucosal surface of the lacrimal passages, which may lead to cicatrization in the lacrimal system. Cicatrization also produces trichiasis, entropion, and dryness of the eye; changes which may lead to corneal damage and loss of vision.

Susceptibility is general; there is no evidence that infection confers immunity. In endemic areas, children have active disease more frequently than adults. Complications increase the longer the disease is present.

The distribution of trachoma is worldwide with a high prevalence in developing and underdeveloped parts of the world including the Middle East, Asia, Africa and South America. The World Health Organization estimates that over 400 million people are infected — of whom 200 million are partially blind and six million are totally blind.

In the Middle East, trachoma is highly prevalent. It is estimated that of the 250 million inhabitants of the Middle East, about 100 million are affected by trachoma.[1] Acquired blindness is a major health problem in the Middle East and trachoma remains the major cause of preventable blindness.[1]

Many epidemiological variables are important in determining the prevalence and intensity of trachoma; climate, cultural patterns, nutrition, trauma and the presence of other infections. However, poor personal hygiene and adverse environmental conditions are the most important factors influencing the disease.

HISTORY OF TRACHOMA IN SAUDI ARABIA

In 1949, Marett,[2] a base surgeon at Dhahran, wrote -

"Saudi Arabia, although showing signs of awakening under the impetus of the new-found oil fields, is still a primitive country[*]. Trachoma or granular conjunctivitis is quite common... the most frequent complications are corneal ulceration, lid deformities, and blindness. There are many blind Arabs but, more often than not, only one eye is blind. Aside from spread due to the close contact with infected persons, the poor nutritional status, bad hygienic surroundings, and the irritant action of the hot desert winds and sands were predisposing factors. The little girls became infected more easily because they attempted to keep cleaner than the boys and the communal use of towels transferred the disease from one to another."

Ten years later, in 1954, a joint program of Trachoma Research was initiated by the Saudi Government, Aramco (Arabian American Oil Company), and the Harvard University School of Public Health.[3] The program was concerned with trachoma and other eye diseases and its principal objectives were the development of more accurate diagnostic methods, the classification of etiology and the attempt to establish means for prevention — including an anti-trachoma vaccine. The program had two laboratories — one in Dhahran, the Eastern Province and the other in Boston. Over 22 years the program generated more than 75 publications

---

[*] Lack of understand of the culture, *(author)*

and a wealth of knowledge which contributed worldwide to the better understanding of trachoma.[4]

Active trachoma and bacterial conjunctivitis were found to be highly prevalent especially in Al-Hasa and the Qatif Oases.[5,6] Conjunctival scraping of 1,200 specimens from Saudi patients in the Eastern Province were examined and revealed 65 strains of adenoviruses, four main species of bacteria (diplococcus, diphtheriod, streptococcus and Koch-Weeks bacillus) and 11 strains of elementary bodies.[3] The main problem was to determine the role of adenoviruses, bacteria and elementary bodies acting alone or in concert with one another, in producing trachoma. In 1957 the causative organism Chlamydia trachomatis was discovered in China.

There was a marked seasonal incidence in the isolations of adenoviruses: 92% of the 65 strains were obtained during the summer months.[7] A strain of elementary bodies isolated from a trachoma patient in the Hofuf oases was shown to be highly toxic for white mice and gerbils when inoculated intravenously in concentrated suspension.[8] This finding was the first step towards the differentiation of trachoma strains.

Several different serotypes of trachoma strains were found in the eyes of subjects within the confines of a single village in the Eastern Province of Saudi Arabia, which remains the only area in the world where all three serotypes of C. trachomatis (A, C and B) have been detected.[9] The three serotypes were noted to have uneven distribution within individual villages. In simultaneous isolations from 40 children in 29 families, siblings were found to have similar immunotypes in 78% of instances.[9] Because of the poor socioeconomic conditions, cases of trachoma were subjected to repeated insults from bacterial or adenoviral infections or physical trauma which resulted in high prevalence of blindness. The accumulated data suggested that the disabling sequelae of trachoma were not related to the intensity of microbiologic infection but to the duration of infection largely determined by the living conditions.[10]

In Al Mallaha village, 96% of the people suffered from trachoma and only 1% of those examined were free from all eye disease. There was a significant relationship between the severity of the disease and the occupation of the head of the family, the number of persons per sleeping area, age, and availability of electricity and running water in the household.[10, 11] No difference was found in the presence of immunoglobins IgA, IgM, IgG in the eye secretions of a group of Boston and Saudi infants, an indication of lack of immunologic deficiencies in the Saudi infants as a basis for susceptibility to trachoma.[12]

Various clinical studies around the world suggested intrafamiliar spread of trachoma.[13, 14, 15] However, the first laboratory-based investigation of families with trachoma was conducted in the Eastern Province in Saudi Arabia.[16] The familial aggregation of trachoma, regardless of the socio-economic differences between families, strongly suggested that the reservoir of infection lies in the household environment. Sleeping habits whereby several persons share the same mattress and pillow and use of the mother's veil in wiping the eyes of her children maximized the exposure to infection. Transmission by flies, water or air in this setting seemed less likely. Attiah et al.,[17] in Egypt, found the highest prevalence of trachoma in infants during the season of minimal fly population.

In 1969, Nichols et al.[18] published their findings on a field trial of trachoma vaccine in young children in the Eastern Province. The bivalent vaccines, inactivated with formalin, were given to 2,117 children in a controlled study. The administration of the vaccines was correlated with a highly significant reduction in inclusions, 6 months after primary inoculation, leading to the hypothesis that a diminution in organisms shed from the eyes of infected patients after vaccination might assist in interrupting the contagious cycle of the disease. The presence of antibodies in eye secretions was shown to be a sensitive and specific test for active trachoma and suggested as a useful tool in epidemiological studies.[19] Efforts to develop a vaccine are still continuing.

Trachoma was and still is the main eye problem in Saudi Arabia, however other problems prevail. The country was subjected from time to time to epidemics of smallpox with it's consequences on the eyes of the population. The last recorded epidemic was in the 1950s. Epidemic hemorrhagic conjunctivitis (EHC) swept throughout Africa and the Middle East during 1969-1973. At the beginning of 1973, an outbreak of EHC occurred in Jeddah, Saudi Arabia.[20] Fletcher[21] observed a high incidence of pre-senile cataract and binocular anomalies (notably squints) among the population of Saudi Arabia. Badr et al.[22] observed in their study of Qasim that beside the 92% prevalence of trachoma among school children, 7.9% had bacterial conjunctivitis of a mild degree.

CURRENT STATUS: THE 1980S

Several studies on trachoma in Saudi Arabia have been conducted in the last 20 years. Table 1 shows the results of some recent surveys.

From the table it is apparent that trachoma is endemic in Saudi Arabia. It affects people living in villages and oases more than city dwellers or nomadic Bedouins. As most of the field studies were conducted among schoolboys, it is only presumed that trachoma is equally prevalent among schoolgirls (Ministry of Health - personal communication).

A change in the severity of the disease and its complications has been noticed. Trachoma, in most cases, does not present the classical picture of large follicles, well developed pannus and thick scar tissue. Instead the follicles are small, corneal vascularization is minimal and little conjunctival scarring occurs.[2] Possible explanations are discussed below.

In the Al Majmaah survey of 766 schoolboys,[23] the clinical diagnosis according to the WHO classification[24] revealed a mean prevalence of trachoma stage I, 94%; stage II, 77%; stage III, 16.4% and stage IV, 3.3%. Similar results of mild trachoma were noticed in Qasim; trachoma stage I, 92%; and trachoma stage IV, 5.3% (Fig. 1).[22]

The role of trachoma as a cause of blindness has also changed. In the 1960s, in Al Mallaha village in Qatif, trachoma was the major cause of blindness. It resulted in the blindness of 26 individuals out of the 406 examined (6.5%).[7]

In 1981, a study of the causes of blindness among 219 blind teachers and students in the Eastern Province[25] showed that ocular infection was responsible for over 70% of the blindness; smallpox 39%, (the history of infection of the youngest victim coincided with the last known smallpox epidemic in the area), bacterial infection 27%, trachoma 3% and toxoplasmosis 1%. Congenital anomalies were responsible for blindness in 16% of the cases. The studied group was mostly of young to middle-aged

---

Table 1. Results of Surveys of Trachoma in Saudi Arabia

First Author	Year of Publication	Ref.	Location	Subjects	% Affected
			Eastern Province		
Nichols	1967	(10)	villages	Pre-school children	90%
			towns	Pre-School children	70%

Fenwick	1980	(11)	Al Mallaha	406 people	96%
Badr	1981	(23)	Majmaah	766 schoolboys	94%
Badr	1984	(22)	Qasim	570 schoolboys	92%
				Bedouin community	80%

persons who became blind in the first 3 years of life whereas trachoma usually causes blindness at a later age. The study does not represent the whole spectrum of blind people.

The study of a group of blind students in Riyadh (1985)[26] also gave an indication of the changing pattern of childhood blindness in Saudi Arabia in the last 20 years. There was a decrease in the acquired causes of blindness and a relative increase in the incidence of genetically determined causes (Tables 2, 3).

In their study in Qasim, Badr *et al.*[22] observed that in older persons in the Kingdom serious visual loss in childhood was due to disease causing ocular damage e.g. perforated corneal ulcers and intraocular infection from neglected bacterial ulcers, and smallpox. In contrast, not a single case due to

Figure 1. Prevalence of Trachoma in 570 Schoolchildren Qasim (1980)

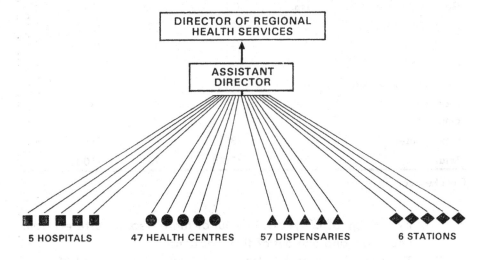

From Ref. 22

these causes was found among schoolchildren and only one child had lost vision through trauma.

Such a change in the severity and sequelae of trachoma in Saudi Arabia could be attributed to the improvement in the standards of living and environmental sanitation as well as the availability of medical care.

A national survey of eye diseases and blindness was conducted in 1984 and covered 16,810 subjects. The highlights but not the detailed results of this survey have been published.[27] Some are given below.

Table 2. Acquired Cases of Childhood Blindness in Saudi Arabia.

Acquired Cases	Born before 1962		Born in or after 1962	
	No.	(%)	No.	(%)
Bacterial keratitis	25	(56)	4	(33)
Smallpox	16	(36)	0	(0)
Accidents	2	(4)	7	(58)
Other	2	(4)	1	(8)
Total	**45**	**(100)**	**12**	**(100)**

From Ref. 26.

Table 3. Genetic Disorders Among 106 Blind Students in Riyadh.

Genetic Disorders	Born before 1962		Born in or after 1962	
	No.	(%)	No.	(%)
Congenital cataract	6	(38)	30	(33)
Primary pigmentary degeneration	1	(6)	26	(29)
Congenital glaucoma	4	(25)	14	(16)
Leber's congenital amaurosis	—		7	(8)
Other causes	5	(39)	13	(15)
Total	**16**	**(100)**	**90**	**(100)**

From Ref. 26.

1. By the age of 60 years, two out of three people suffered from visual loss and one out of five was blind.
2. The prevalence of blindness was 1.5% of the population by WHO standards (Visual Acuity of less than 3/60 in the better eye with the best correction). If the USA standard was taken (Visual Acuity less than 6/60), the blindness rate became 2.6%.

This compared unfavorably with the rate of 0.1 to 0.3% in Western countries.

3.   Visual impairment and blindness increased dramatically with age.

4.   Blindness was found more frequently in females than in males at all ages.

5.   The leading causes of blindness were:

Cataract	55.1%
Trachoma	10.1%
Corneal scars	9.1%
Refractive errors	9.0%
Failure of treatment	4.7%
Glaucoma	3.0%

It is evident that most of the causes of blindness are avoidable and they could have been prevented or cured at an early stage.

Research programs in the field of eye diseases are active, and the King Khalid Eye Specialist Hospital in Riyadh plays a leading role. Among the research programs currently undertaken are ocular manifestations of bejel and yaws, climatic droplet keratopathy, conjunctival shrinkage caused by home-made remedies, causes of bacterial corneal ulcers, the health care perceptions of Saudi women, and others.[28]

CONTROL

The objectives of a trachoma control program should be the reduction of both the prevalence and severity of the disease. The strategy to achieve such an objective involves several components:

1.   Improving basic medical education by integrating clinical opthalmology with community medicine.

2.   Training of opthalmologists and optometrists. It has been estimated that 30 members of each category need to be trained annually.[27]

3.   Family physicians and other members of the health team at the level of primary health care, if well trained, can play a significant role by providing comprehensive health care and

improving awareness among the public regarding the etiology of the disease and its relation to personal hygiene. A sense of responsibility among the community can be successfully developed.[29]

4. Health education on personal hygiene.

5. Religious concepts in health education should be used effectively "He (God) loves those who keep themselves pure and clean."[30] "When you prepare for prayer wash your faces and your hands to elbows, wipe your head and wash your feet to the ankle."[31]

6. A trachoma campaign should start with baseline data to plan for the control and monitor progress. Both clinical and laboratory methods should be used.

7. Mass treatment for whole families should be administered in areas of high prevalence. The drug of choice is oxytetracycline ointment once or twice daily for a week each month for 6 months.

In conclusion the prevalence rate of trachoma is still high (in the range of 70-80%) in the communities which have been studied and the people affected are still at the risk of visual reduction. *Chlamydia trachomatis* infection in Saudi Arabia is largely ocular, as compared to genital infection which is more usual in Western societies. The problem of trachoma and other eye diseases in Saudi Arabia may be partly solved by socioeconomic development, but maximally successful control needs planned action.

REFERENCES

1. **Majcuk J.** Trachoma control in the Eastern Mediterranean Region. *WHO Chron* 1976; 30: 97-100.

2. **Marret WC.** Some medical problems in Saudi Arabia. *US Armed Forces Med J 1953; 4: 31-38.*

3. **Page RC.** Progress report on the Aramco trachoma research programme. *Med Bull Standard Oil Co. (NJ)* 1959; 19: 68-73.

4. **Nichols RL** ed. *Trachoma research program: chlamydial research publications.* Dhahran, Saudi Arabia: Aramco/Boston, Massachusetts, USA: Harvard School of Public Health (1954-1981); 1982.

5. **Snyder JC, Page RC, Murray ES** *et al.* Observations on the etiology of trachoma. *Am J Opthalmol* 1959; 48: 325-329.

6. **Hanna AT.** *The epidemiology of trachoma and conjunctival infections in a Saudi Arabian oasis.* Harvard School of Public Health, Mass., USA: Department of Epidemiology. September, 1959. Doctoral thesis.

7. **Nichols RL, McComb DE, Snyder JC.** Chlamydia trachomatis infections of the eye in the Eastern Province of Saudi Arabia: a review of 21 years of research. In: *Proceedings of the 4ᵗʰ Saudi Medical Conference.* Dammam: King Faisal University, 1980: 77-103.

8. **Murray ES, Snyder JC, Bell SD Jr.** A note on the toxicity or white mice and gerbilles of a strain of elementary bodies isolated from a patient with trachoma in Eastern Saudi Arabia. In: *Proc 6ᵗʰ Int Congr Trop Med Malaria* 1958; 5: 530-535.

9. **Nichols RL, Von Fritzinger K, McComb DE,** Epidemiological data derived from immunotyping of **338** trachoma strains isolated from children in Saudi Arabia. In: Nichols RL (ed). *Trachoma and related disorders caused by chlamydial agents.* Amsterdam: Excerpta Medica, 1971; Series 223: 337-357.

10. **Nichols RL, Bobb AA, Haddad NA, McComb DE.** Immunofluorescence studies of the microbiological epidemiology of trachoma in Saudi Arabia. *Am J Opthalmol 1967; 63: 1371-1442.*

11. **Fenwick SA, McComb DE, Allen HF, Oertley RE, Nichols RL.** Catastrophic visual disabilities in Saudi Arabian villagers. Association of holoendemic trachoma, socio-economic factors and severity of disease sequellae, including blindness. (Submitted for publication).

12. **Mull JD, Peters JH, Nichols RL.** Immunoglobins, secretory component, and transferrin in eye secretions of infants in regions with and without endemic trachoma. *Infect Immun* 1970; 2: 489-494.

13. **Foster SO.** Trachoma in American Indian village. *Pub Hlth Rep* 1965; 80: 829-832.

14. **Taylor CE, Gulati PV, Harinarian J.** Eye infections in a Punjab village. *Am J Trop Med Hyg* 1958; 7: 42-50.

15. **Haddad NA.** Trachoma in Lebanon: observations on epidemiology in rural areas. *Am J Trop Med Hyg 1965; 14: 652-653.*

16. **Barenfanger J.** Studies on the role of the family unit in the transmission of trachoma. *Am J Trop Med Hyg* 1975; 24: 509-515.

17. **Attiah MAH, El Kholy AM, Omran AR.** Epidemiological pattern of initial trachoma infection in a rural community in UAR. *J Egypt Med Ass* 1962; 45: 623-637

18. **Nichols RL, Bell SD Jr., Haddad NA, Bobb AA.** Studies on trachoma: VI: microbiological observations in a field trial in Saudi Arabia of bivalent trachoma vaccine at three dosage levels. *Am J Trop Med Hyg* 1969; 18: 723-730.

19. **McComb DE, Nichols RL.** Antibodies to trachoma in eye secretions of Saudi Arab children. *Am J Epidemiol* 1969; 90: 278-284.

20. **Maitchouk I,** Epidemic haemorrhagic conjunctivitis pandemic of a new type of virus eye disease. *WHO/EM/VIR/4* 1972: 18 pp.

21. **Fletcher RJ, Voke J.** The need for eye correction training in Saudi Arabia. *Saudi Med J* 1982; 3: 119-123.

22. **Badr I, Qureshi I.** Ocular status of schoolchildren in Al Asiah Qasim Region. In: Sebai Z.A. ed. *Community health in Saudi Arabia: a profile of two villages in Qasim Region,* 2nd ed. Jeddah: Tihama Publications, 1984: 24-27.

23. **Badr I, Qureshi I.** Ocular status of school children in the town of Al-Majma'ah, Central Province, Saudi Arabia. *Saudi Med J* 1981; 2: 221-224.

24. Expert committee on trachoma (third report) World Health Organization. *Tech Rep Ser* 1962; 234: 15-19.

25. **Badr IA, Qureshi IH.** Cause of blindness in the Eastern Province of blind schools. *Saudi Med J* 1983; 4: 331-338.

26. **Tabbara KF, Badr IA.** Changing pattern of childhood blindness in Saudi Arabia. *Br J Opthalmol* 1985; 69: 312-315.

27. **Tabbara KF, Badr IA, Paton D, Ross-Degnan D, Meaders R.** Survey of eye disease and blindness in the Kingdom of Saudi Arabia. *Opthalmology* 1984; 91: 141.

28. **Tabbara** KF. *Quarterly Report.* Research Department, Riyadh, Saudi Arabia: King Khalid Eye Specialist Hospital. 30th September 1984.

29. **Sebai Z.A.** Introduction to Qasim project. In: Sebai Z.A. ed. *Community Health in Saudi Arabia. A profile of two villages in Qasim Region,* 2nd ed. Jeddah: Tihama Publications, 1984: 1-10.
30. **Quran,** *Surat II Al-Bagara* (The Cow) verse 222.
31. **Quran,** *Surat V Al-Maaidah* (The Table) verse 6.

NUTRITIONAL DISORDERS

Up to 25% of the infants born in developing countries have a birth weight of less than 2,500 grams. They are subjected to malnutrition during their intrauterine life, and throughout their childhood. Depletion of maternal resources, lack of maternity care, poverty and ignorance are contributing factors to this problem. Malnutrition can be primary (exogenous) or secondary (endogenous), and a result of overnutrition or undernutrition. It ranges from mild retardation of growth or being slightly overweight to severe protein-energy malnutrition or obesity.

In children, malnutrition interacts with entrocolitis and respiratory infection. The triad is the leading cause of morbidity and mortality among pre-school children in the developing world.

INTRODUCTION

Several studies (none at a national or regional level) have been conducted on selected groups of people in Saudi Arabia (employees, pre-school children and hospital patients) to define their nutritional status.

In general, an improvement in the nutritional status of the Saudis has been observed over the last two decades. This is a repercussion of socioeconomic development and improvement in education, dietary habits, and environmental conditions.

One of the earliest studies on nutritional problems was among Aramco (Arabian American Oil Company) employees in 1957.[1] Their average diet showed 28% deficiency in proteins, 72% in fat and 5% in carbohydrates, compared to a standard, 2,800 calorie, balanced diet. The study also revealed that 39% of the surveyed group (number not provided) were more than 15% underweight by American standards. It is however very dubious to what extent the norms from one ethnic group are applicable to another. The low levels of serum protein and the high incidence of enlarged livers (27.7%) were also attributed to nutritional deficiencies. Arteriosclerosis was seldom seen.

The findings, in the opinion of the researchers, were due to long-standing nutritional deficiencies rather than any inherent characteristic of the race. Although the study lacked many scientific merits, it revealed a problem of malnutrition among a selected sector of the population.

Several researchers were interested in the anthropometric measurements and the clinical assessments of pre-school children. Such indices reflect the health status of the community.

In 1967 Sebai[2] conducted a field survey to study the health and nutritional status of pre-school children in Turaba, a rural community in the Western Region. Out of 332 children examined clinically, 21 (6%) had one or more positive clinical signs of malnutrition. Their weights and heights were significantly lower than the 50th percentile of a standard reference.

Figure 1. Nutritional status of 827 children in three rural communities in Saudi Arabia.

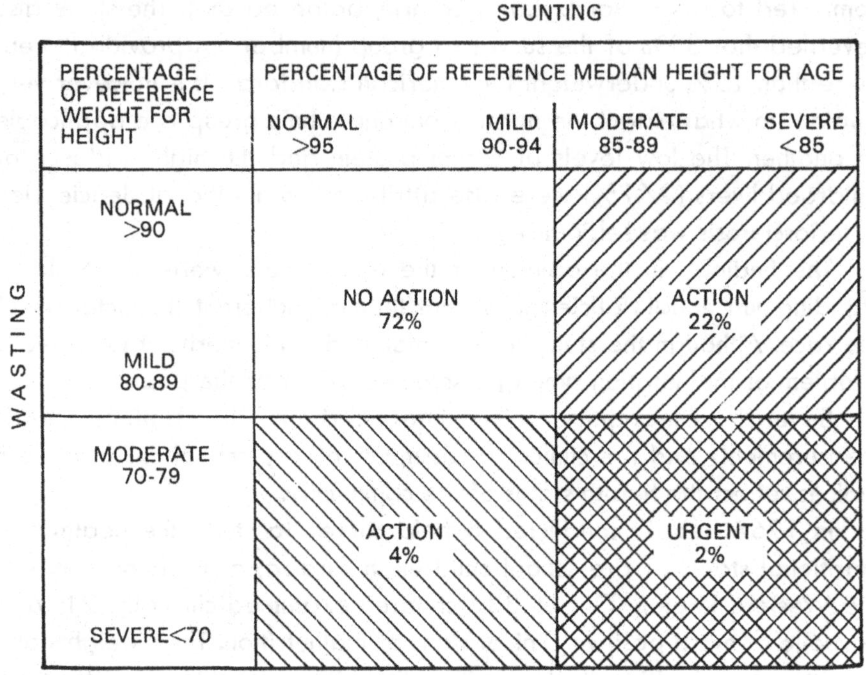

STUNTING

PERCENTAGE OF REFERENCE WEIGHT FOR HEIGHT	PERCENTAGE OF REFERENCE MEDIAN HEIGHT FOR AGE			
	NORMAL >95	MILD 90-94	MODERATE 85-89	SEVERE <85
NORMAL >90 ... MILD 80-89	NO ACTION 72%		ACTION 22%	
MODERATE 70-79 ... SEVERE<70	ACTION 4%		URGENT 2%	

WASTING

Source: Ref. 4.

In 1978 two studies were carried out on the nutritional status of children in three communities; Tamnia, the coastal land of Tihama, and a Bedouin community in the Central Region.[3,4] Figure 1 summarizes the anthropometric measurements of 827 pre-school children in the three communities: 72% were either normal or mildly affected, 26% had a mild-to-moderate degree of stunting or wasting (required action) and 2% were severely wasted and stunted (needing an urgent action).

Of 279 children examined clinically in Tamnia, two were marasmic, one had rickets and 91 children (36%) were anemic. The cause of enlarged liver found in 10 children was presumed, in the absence of malaria and schistosomiasis, to be nutritional. No other clinical signs of drastic malnutrition or vitamin deficiency were seen.

Hammam[5] carried out a nutritional survey of 317 schoolboys and 153 schoolgirls in Barza, a rural community in Western Saudi Arabia in 1978. He found that 57.1% of the boys and 32.0% of the girls in the age group 6-18 years fell below the third percentile of American children of the same age group. Again the reason behind the differences could be partly ethnic and partly environmental.

In 1980 a health survey was conducted in rural Qasim.[6] On clinical examination of 337 children only two marasmus, one kwashiorkor, two angular stomatitis and three rickets cases were detected. Height and weight measurements compared to the Harvard Standard showed that 82.8% were either normal or had a mild degree of malnutrition; 16.3% had moderate stunting or wasting, and 0.9% had severe stunting or wasting and required urgent action.

Wirths[7] studied 341 students in Riyadh, Jeddah, Abha and Dammam. The Saudi boys were found to be smaller and leaner than boys from the USA, Europe, other Arabian countries and well-to-do Indian boys.

Humeida[8] evaluated the birth weight length and head circumference of 400 (200 males and 200 females) normal, full-term Saudi newborns in King Abdul Aziz University Hospital in Jeddah. The medium birth weight of the Saudi infants were 3.27 kg. It was significantly less than the medium birth weight of North American infants (3.42 kg), but compared favorably to the Northern Nigerian infants (3.02 kg), Indians (3.10 kg) and West Indians (3.22 kg).

Table 1 lists the ten most common causes of admission of 5,788 children under 12 years of age to the Children's Hospital, Riyadh, in a 3-month period in 1981.[9] Nutritional deficiencies are low on the list but they are, obviously, a cause of the high percentage of admissions for respiratory disorders and entrocolitis.

In all of these surveys, except one, the anthropometric measurements showed a mild-to-moderate degree of stunting and wasting compared to international figures. Very few signs of severe malnutrition or gross vitamin deficiencies were elicited in these or other studies.[10, 11] However, one has to consider not only ethnic differences in such comparative studies but also differences in methods used in data collection and analysis.

The hemoglobin level was another interesting health index for researchers. In the Turaba study conducted in 1967[2] 34% of the Bedouin children were anemic (10 g %). In 1968 McNeil[12] studied infants and children who attended the well-baby clinic in Aramco Hospital, Dhahran. Of the 500 children examined, 198 (39.6%) were anemic, mostly because of inadequate dietary iron. Over a period of 2 years, 100 of the anemic children were followed-up; 82% had again developed anemia, mostly due to iron deficiency.

In the Tamnia study in 1978,[3] 36% of the children were anemic. Sejeny[13] in 1978 examined 527 anemic patients in the King Abdul Aziz Hospital in Jeddah, 50.4% of whom were normochromic, 47.4% hypochromic and 2.2% macrocytic. The causes of anemia were infections, blood loss and pregnancy among females. Only one case of B12 deficiency was found.

The study conduced by Hafez[14] among 48 primary care patients in Riyadh, although of a small scale, showed some interesting features:

1. Causes of anemia in the group studied were different from those in Western societies. Whereas 67% of cases in the group studied were caused by iron deficiency (Table 2), the figure in Britain is 91%.[15]

2. Iron-deficiency anemia is frequently encountered among females, especially in the child-bearing age group.

3. Over a 3-year period, no megaloblastic anemia was found among primary care patients of the Riyadh Armed Forces Hospital.

In 1982 a survey was carried out among 217 pregnant Saudi women at the Jeddah Armed Forces Hospital to investigate their hemoglobin levels.[16] Only 14 women had hemoglobins below 10g/dl at some stage in pregnancy. The Saudi diet seems to be as adequate as a standard Western diet for pregnancy. The findings were comparable to those among 436 pregnant Saudi women studied in Asir (altitude of 2,133.6 m [7000 feet]) where only 5% were anemic (<10 g/dl).[17] However, the two studies were carried out among selected groups of the population (the Armed Forces dependents).

Anemia, mostly iron deficiency, is apparently a common problem among the studied groups. Consideration, however, should be given to the possible

---

Table 1. Admissions to the Children's Hospital - Shemaisi, Riyadh over 3 months (January - March 1981).

Main causes of admission (WHO) classification)	Admission (%)
Respiratory disorders:	
Lower tract, e.g. pneumonia, asthma	30.8
Upper tract, e.g. tonsillitis, coryza, etc.	30.1

Intestinal disorders:	
Gastroenteritis, etc.	20.1
Appendix, hernia, etc.	2.1
Blood disorders:	
Anemia, sickle cell disease	4.3
Accidental poisoning: Drugs, kerosene	4.2
Ear, nose and throat disorders:	2.2
Bacterial disorders:	
Pertussis, tetanus, tuberculosis	2.2
Viral diseases:	
Measles, poliomyelitis	2.1
CNS diseases:	
Meningitis, epilepsy, cerebral palsy	2.1
Perinatal conditions	1.9
Nutritional deficiencies: Rickets, marasmus	1.7
Total no. of admitted under 12 years of age	5,788
Total no. of diagnoses	6,785
Average no. of diagnoses per child	1.2

From Ref. 9

differences in physiological norms between Saudis and other populations before making a final judgment.

Rickets was never known to be a problem in Saudi Arabia until Elidrissy published his study in 1980.[18] He reported 31 cases of vitamin-D deficiency rickets who were admitted to the Riyadh Maternity and Children's Hospital over a period of 14 months (1979-1980). They consisted of 18 males and 13 females (2 - 24 months) of low socioeconomic status who mostly presented in the winter season with respiratory symptoms. Elidrissy attributed these unexpected findings, in the sunny climate of Arabia, to the limited exposure of babies to sunshine as a result of the habit of overdressing them and keeping them in-doors in badly illuminated houses. Continued breast feeding for a long period without supplementary food was found to be another factor. The author concluded that infantile rickets is underdiagnosed in Saudi Arabia and the cases that came to his notice were but the 'tip of the iceberg'.

Table 2. Type of Anemia Among 48 Patients From Riyadh Armed Services
Hospital.

	Males	Females	Total
Iron Deficiency	8	24	32
G-6-PD	3	0	3
Beta Thalassemia Minor	4	2	6
Beta Thalassemia Major	0	1	1
Sickle Trait (S/A)	2	3	5
Sickle Disease (S/S)	1	0	1
Megaloblastic	0	0	0

From: Ref. 14

The results of the Elidrissy's study encouraged Sedrani[19] to investigate the status of vitamin D in a sample of 175 people living in Riyadh for more than 2 years. The study showed that a high proportion (up to 53%) of the sample had low serum 25 hydroxyvitamin D concentration (below 10 ng/ml). In another study Sedrani et al.[20] found that the average dietary vitamin D intake of Saudis is 55iu/day which is approximately one-seventh of that recommended in the USA. The level of the dihydroxylated vitamin D metabolites, namely 1,25- and 24, 25-dihydroxy cholecalciferol, was normal in a sample of male university students but deficient in elderly persons.

The authors suggested that the low vitamin D3 status in the elderly Saudi population is mainly due to the avoidance of sunlight, dietary vitamin D deficiency and an increase in ultraviolet light insulation due to atmospheric dust particles. The clothing style of the Saudi population was excluded as a possible cause since adequate serum 25-(OH) D3 levels have been found in female students who veiled themselves and were more extensively clothed. The authors called for fortification of milk and milk products with vitamin D and modification of housing design to admit more sunlight.

Elidrissy et al.[21] studied 74 rachitic and non-rachitic children and their interpretation was that after the first 6 months of life, the vitamin D content of breast milk is inadequate to prevent rickets. Infants need supplementary vitamin D and more exposure to sunlight. Further studies are suggested to define the normal physiological values of vitamin D, and the magnitude and etiology of the problem.

The study of dietary habits of the Saudi family, especially infants, was the focus of interest for some field workers.[22, 23] Sebai, 15 years after his initial study in Turaba, found that many mothers shifted from breast to artificial feeding of their infants.[2] This attitude was also evident in the studies carried out recently in Tamnia[3] and Qasim.[6, 24] Artificial feeding of infants has become a sign of modernization.

In 1981 Lawson[25] observed that many infants and young children seen at Riyadh Military hospital had nutritional disorders and that there was a "dearth of published information on child rearing practices in the Arabian Peninsula. Malnutrition was due to decreased breast feeding, poor hygiene and inappropriate weaning practice." She identified 31 brands of milk in Riyadh market. When mothers were asked about the reasons for giving supplementary feeds, the majority mentioned inadequate, or lack of, breast milk. A pregnant woman's milk is believed to be poisonous to the baby and is a common reason for terminating breast feeding. Figure 2 shows the feeding patterns during the first year of life among infants attending Riyadh Military Hospital.

Elias[26] also found that 70% of mothers attending the primary health care clinic in the Military Hospital in Taif start by breast feeding and end by bottle — or mixed feeding by the end of the first year. She observed 12 different brands of formula feed on sale in Taif. "Some of these brands were unsuitable because they contained starch, sugar or excessive sodium anions and would not have been permitted for sale in the USA or Britain".

Rahman[27] found, by interviewing 560 Saudi women, that 81% believed that breast feeding was the easiest and the most nutritious method of infant feeding. Such were the mothers' attitudes, but in practice and at the time of survey, only 63% of the mothers actually breast fed their infants, 11% used bottle feeding and 26% used mixed feeding.

There is a difference in opinion as to the influence of the change in dietary habits on the health of the people. Sebai[2] attributed the apparent improvement in the health status of Turaba children to the improvement of the family's economic power to purchase food and the growing awareness of nutritional values.

Hamidi[28] compared the old and newly emerging dietary patterns in rural Saudi Arabia. She suggested that the traditional family menu consisting of locally produced food; dates, *markook* (cooked vegetables and a wholewheat pasta), *kursan* (cooked vegetables and wholewheat wafers), and milk, is more nutritious than new diets consisting of white unenriched bread, rice, jam, cheese, sugar etc. She made her point clear "Dietary change is rapid, radical and in need of guidance from trained personnel".

DISCUSSION

This review of the literature on nutritional disorders in Saudi Arabia indicates that our information is still inadequate. The number of works published in the last decade exceeds what has been published before in total, which is a promising sign. The studies referred to were conducted among selected populations; small villages, nomadic communities, company employees or hospital patients; none were representative of a region or the nation.

Most of the studies revealed problems of anemia and mild-to-moderate degrees of stunting and wasting among pre-school children. The causes are, apparently, ignorance and misconception rather than being purely economical. Recently, overnutrition has been observed as a problem among the middle and upper classes of urban societies.

On the basis of the fieldwork there is no proof that severe nutritional disorders are a problem in Saudi Arabia. Collectively, out of 948 pre-school children surveyed in Turaba, Tamnia, and Qasim only six had *kwashiorkor* and four had

Figure 2: Infant feeding pattern, Riyadh (1980)

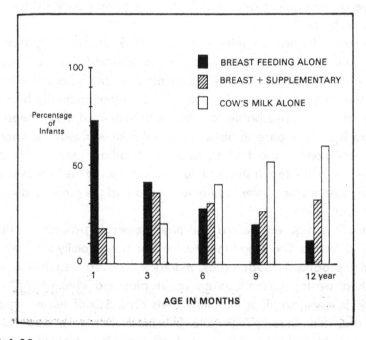

From: Ref. 25.

marasmus. No cases of beriberi, pellagra or vitamin A deficiencies were reported. Among the ten main causes of admission to the Children's Hospital in Riyadh, malnutrition came low on the list, although it may well be a contributing factor to the high rate of respiratory diseases and gastroenteritis.

The unexpected discovery of 31 cases of rickets in 1980 drew the attention of several researchers to the problem. Saudis are inadequately exposed to sunlight and their food has an insufficient content of vitamin D.

Some field surveys have been conducted to describe the dietary habits of small communities. Although rice and bread are the staple foods in rural areas, the improvement of purchasing power and a better awareness of the nutritional values have brought varieties of foods, both local and imported, to the family menu.

Artificial infant feeding, with its subsequent hazards, has become a sign of modernization in urban and rural communities. Solid food is introduced late during infancy and is not always nutritious.

Most of the studies have used standard foreign references for comparing results. Before final judgment can be made, one has to consider racial and ethnic variances between the compared groups. A national survey is needed to assess the problem of malnutrition in Saudi Arabia and its etiological factors and to design a strategy for its control.

WHICH WAY FORWARD?

1. Our knowledge of the nutritional problems in Saudi Arabia is still inadequate. National, regional and local nutritional surveys are needed. The survey results should not end as documents kept in files or on shelves but rather as initiators for action. They should serve as tools for planning, evaluation and feedback.

2. The problem of anemia and mild-to-moderate degrees of stunting and wasting among pre-school children, as revealed by the field studies are, apparently, due to ignorance and misconception rather than economical. Health education programs should be expanded and improved in content and methods. The best approaches would be through person to person contacts, group discussions and community involvement. Primary Health Care units are the most appropriate places for such actions. Mass media also should have an active role.

3.   The rapid process of urbanization, settlement and contacts with the outside world led to fast socioeconomical changes and changes in behaviour and life styles of city dwellers, villagers and nomadic Bedouins. These changes bring along with them health hazards such as obesity and artificial feeding for infants. Improving awareness and self-reliance of the people is essential.

4.   The time is ripe to create Saudi standards for health and nutrition. These are to be used as yardsticks for planning and evaluation of health and nutritional programs.

REFERENCES

1.   **Page RC.** Practical aspects of employee nutrition. *Indust and Trop Hlth* 1957; 3: 120-127.

2.   **Sebai ZA.** *The health of the family in a changing Arabia.* 3rd ed. Jeddah: Tihama Publications, 1983: 155 pp.

3.   **Sebai ZA, El Hazmi MAF, Serenius F.** Health profile of preschool children in Tamnia villages, Saudi Arabia. In: *Priorities in Child Care. Saudi Med J* 1981; 2 (Suppl 1): 68-71.

4.   **Serenies F. Fougerouse D.** Health and nutritional status in rural Saudi Arabia. In: *Priorities in Child Care. Saudi Med J* 1981; 2 (Suppl 1): 10-22.

5.   **Hammam HM, Kamel LM, Hidayat NM.** A health profile of a rural community in the western zone of Saudi Arabia. In: *Proceedings of the 4th Saudi Medical Conference.* Dammam: King Faisal University, 1980: 26-34.

6.   **Abdulla MA, Sebai ZA, Swailem AR.** Health and nutritional status of preschool children. In: Sebai ZA. ed. *Community Health in Saudi Arabia: a profile of two villages in Qasim Region. Saudi Med J,* Monogr No. 1 2nd ed Jeddah: Tihama Publications, 1985: 11-18.

7.   **Wirths W, Hamdan M, Hayati M, Rajhi H.** Ernahrungsstatus, nahrungsverbrauch und nahrstoffzufuhr von schulern in Saudi Arabian: Anthropometriche Daten. *Zeitshrift fur Ernahrungswissenschaft* 1977; 16:1-11.

8.   **Humeida AK, Hardy MJ.** Birth weights, occipito-frontal circumferences and crown to heel lengths in four-hundred normal, healthy Saudi Babies. In: Mahjoub ES, *et al.* eds. *Proceedings*

of the *5th Saudi Medical Meeting.* Riyadh: University of Riyadh, 1981: 419-427.

9. **Laurance BM.** What can be done to keep Saudi children healthy? *Saudi Med J* 1982; 3: 221-224.

10. **Hassan MM.** Multiple nutritional deficiencies and multiple infections. *King Abdulaziz Med J* 1982; 2: 51-58.

11. **Mohamed AE, Madkour MM.** Pernicious anemia in a Saudi male. *Saudi Med J* 1984; 5: 201-203.

12. **McNiel JR.** Variation in the response of childhood iron deficiency anemia to oral iron. *Blood* 1968; 31: 641-646.

13. **Sejeny SA, Khurshid M, Kamil A, Khan FA.** Anemia survey in the southwestern region of Saudi Arabia. In: *Proceedings of the 4th Saudi Medical Conference,* Dammam: King Faisal University 1980: 124-128.

14. **Hafez A. Marshall I.** A survey of anemia from June 1981 to January 1982 in the Department of Primary Care, Riyadh Al-Kharj Hospital Programme. In: *Proceedings of the 7th Saudi Medical Meeting,* Dammam: King Faisal University, 503-505.

15. **Fry J.** *Common diseases - their natural incidence and care.* 2nd edition Lancaster MTP Press Ltd, 1979: 209.

16. **Smart Sm, Duncan ME, Kalina JM.** Haemoglobin levels and anemia in pregnant Saudi women. *Saudi Med J* 1983; 4: 263-268.

17. **Hartley DRW.** One thousand obstetric deliveries in the Asir Province, Kingdom of Saudi Arabia: A Review. *Saudi Med J* 1980; 1: 187-196.

18. **Elidrissy ATH, Taha SA.** Rickets in Riyadh. In: Mahgoub ES, *et al.* eds. *Proceedings of the 5th Saudi Medical Meeting.* Riyadh: University of Riyadh, 1981: 409-418.

19. **Sedrani SH.** Low 25-hydroxyvitamin D and normal serum calcium concentration in Saudi Arabia: Riyadh Region. *Ann Nutrit Metab* 1984; 28: 181-185.

20. **Sedrani SH, Elidrissy ATH, El Arabi KM.** Sunlight and vitamin D status in normal Saudi subjects. *Am J Clin Nutr* 1983; 38: 129-132.

21. **Elidrissy ATH, El Swailem AR, Belton NR, Aldress AZ, Forfar JO.** 25-hydroxy vitamin D in rachitic, non-rachitic and marasmus children in Saudi Arabia. In: *Vitamin D, chemical, biochemical and*

clinical endocrinology of calcium metabolism. Berlin-New York: Walter de Gruyter & Co, 1982: 617-619.

22. Anonymous. Medical, nutritional and social study of sample of Riyadh schoolgirls Department of Nutrition, Ministry of Health-1977: (Arabic).

23. Anonymous. Results of a field survey on health, nutrition and social welfare of preschool children in Riyadh, Department of Nutrition, Ministry of Health 1981: (Arabic).

24. **Sebai ZA, Shalaby EME.** The family setting. In: Sebai ZA. ed. *Community health in Saudi Arabia: a profile of two villages in Qasim Region. Saudi Med J*, Monog No. 1, 2nd ed. Jeddah: Tihama Publications, 1985; 35-40.

25. **Lawson M.** Infant feeding Habits in Riyadh. In: *Priorities in Child Care. Saudi Med J* 1981; 2 (Suppl 1): 26-29.

26. **Elias JBT.** A survey of place of delivery, modes of milk feeding and immunization in a primary health care centre in Saudi Arabia. *Saudi Med J* 1985; 6: 169-176.

27. **Rahman J, Farrag OA, Chatterjee TK, Rahman MS, Al-Awdah S.** Pattern of infant feeding in the Eastern Province of Saudi Arabia. In: *Proceedings of the 7th Saudi Medical Meeting.* Dammam: King Faisal University, Dammam, 1982; 407-411.

28. **Hamidi E.** A call for clinical dietetic training in the Kingdom of Saudi Arabia. *Saudi Med J* 1981; 2: 44-47.

DIABETES MELLITUS

INTRODUCTION

Knowledge of diabetes dates to centuries before Christ. The Egyptian papyrus Ebers (1500 B.C.) described an illness associated with "the passage of much urine". Celsius (30 B.C. to 50 A.D.) recognized the disease but it was not until two centuries later that another Greek physician, Aretaeus of Cappadocia, gave it the name diabetes (siphon). He made the first clinical description, "a melting down of the flesh and limbs into urine."[1] In 1921 the role of insulin in treating diabetic patients was discovered.

Diabetes mellitus is a relative deficiency of insulin secretion by the pancreas, resulting in the diminished ability of the body to metabolize carbohydrates, frequently associated with disturbances in the metabolism of proteins and fats. The cause is unknown, but obesity, racial susceptibility and heredity are etiologic factors.

There are two common varieties of diabetes, though in reality they form a spectrum of insulin deficiency.

1. Insulin-dependent diabetes mellitus (IDDM or Type 1), a ketosis-prone type of diabetes associated with certain histocompatibility antigens (HLA) controlled by genes on chromosome 6 and with

islet cell antibodies (juvenile onset). It may be related to viral infection.[2]

2.   Non-insulin-dependent diabetes mellitus (NIDDM or Type 2), a non-ketosis-prone type of diabetes not secondary to other diseases or conditions (maturity onset). This subclass of diabetes has been subdivided into obese NIDDM and non-obese NIDDM.[3]

Diabetes tends to be seen in families, is associated with accelerated atherosclerosis, and predisposes to certain specific microvascular abnormalities including retinopathy, nephropathy and neuropathy. It increases the risk of stroke, heart attacks and peripheral vascular problems. Symptoms include polyuria, polydipsia, polyphagia, loss of weight, weakness and pruritus — particularly of the perineum in women.

Obesity requires a higher plasma insulin concentration, therefore, a greater rate of insulin release is needed to control glucose levels. Insulin uptake by cells and insulin effectiveness is thus reduced with obesity and the pancreas must produce larger quantities of insulin. For this reason populations in which diabetes is not a public health problem may show an increased incidence of diabetes as they become more affluent or their carbohydrate intake increases markedly.[4]

The distribution of diabetes varies according to age, sex, cultural differences, dietary patterns and methods of ascertainment and diagnostic criteria. This makes international comparisons rather difficult. The incidence rate of IDDM among children varies from 0.6 per 100,000 per year in Tokyo, Japan to 29 per 100,000 per year in Finland, whereas the incidence rate of IDDM in the age group 40-49 years varies between 2.0 per 1,000 per year among White Americans to 57.0 per 1,000 per year among Puma Indians, Arizona.[5]

According to the WHO Expert Committee on Diabetes Mellitus "Diabetes is a universal health problem affecting human species at all stages of development. It is common in all corpulated and physically inactive populations irrespective of race".[6] The majority of cases of diabetes in the Middle East are of NIDDM.[7] Interactions between heredity and environment including changes in lifestyle, degree of physical activity and availability of food are probably behind the emerging problem of diabetes in the Middle East.[8]

THE PROBLEM IN SAUDI ARABIA

Although diabetes mellitus in Saudi Arabia has attracted the attention of many researchers and several meetings have been held in the past 5 years on the subject, only a few studies have been published. These studies were carried out in local communities and mostly amongst hospital patients.

The presence of glucose in the urine has been used widely in the past to measure diabetes. However, in recent years the validity of this procedure has been questioned. In the Riyadh Military Hospital, a study was carried out among 149 patients to correlate findings on serum and urine glucose in native-born Saudi Arabs.[9] The Saudi diabetics were found to have, on average, higher renal thresholds for glucose than American and European populations. Using clearance urine excretions and midpoint serum glucose assays, 50% of the men and 48% of the women were found not to exhibit glycosuria when their serum glucose was >180 mg/100 ml. Seventy-five per cent of the women and 62% of the men did not have glycosuria when their serum glucose was between 220 and 259 mg/ml. It was concluded that urine testing for control of diabetes is not useful in the majority of Saudi diabetics and control should be assessed by serum glucose measurement.

A study was conducted among 1,385 male and 128 female Saudis in the Al Kharj region to investigate the prevalence of diabetes mellitus.[10, 11] Accessibility to females was difficult. Diabetes was found in 2.5% of the males and 4.7% of the females. In 510 males over 35 years of age, the prevalence rate was 6.5% which is higher than the rate reported in Western countries. Of those who were under 35 years of age (875 males and 71 females) only one male was diabetic. None of the patients admitted having polyuria and polydipsia. However, 65% of the males and all the females were overweight. Biochemical analysis did not reveal a significant occurrence of liver or renal problems.

The conclusion was that diabetes mellitus is relatively common in the Al Kharj Saudi community. It is mainly related to increasing age and obesity. Because of the absence of polyuria and polydipsia among Saudis, screening of the population for diabetes is, therefore, an important measure required to control the problem.

A large overlap in the fasting values of serum glucose in diabetics and normal subjects was found in another study.[12] The suggestion was made that the WHO recommendations were not suitable for interpretation of glucose values in Saudi Arabs. It was felt that reliance on a fasting value for the diagnosis of diabetes is inappropriate in Saudi Arabians and that only the 2h post-glucose assessment should be used for screening the disease.[13]

In contrast to the low prevalence rate of young diabetics in Al Kharj,[11] a study over a period of 12 months in King Abdul Aziz Hospital in Jeddah showed that 13 cases out of 65 in-patient diabetics were under 30 years of age.[14] Three out of the 65 had maturity-onset diabetes of youth (MODY) which is a rare mild non-ketotic form of insulin-dependent juvenile diabetes. The impression given was that diabetes is a common problem among young age groups. However, the sample was too small and selective to lead to generalized conclusions.

Between 1977 and 1982, 11 Saudi Arab children under 14 years of age were diagnosed to have diabetes mellitus among Aramco (Arabian American Oil Company) employees' dependents in the Eastern Province.[15] The incidence rate was 0.7 per 10,000 children per year and the point prevalence was 1 per 5,000 children. The prevalence was less than that reported from many Western countries[16, 17, 18] but similar to that in France where the disease affects one in every 4,200 children under 15 years old.[19] Males predominated in the group (male: female 8:3). Polydipsia with or without polyuria was the common symptom (82%) (differing from the Al Kharj Study[11]). Parental education and compliance with treatment were necessary for the optimal care of these patients.

A study of 222 non-insulin dependent Saudi diabetics in King Faisal Specialist Hospital and Research Center, Riyadh[20] showed some interesting findings. Coronary artery disease, large vessel peripheral vascular disease, retinopathy and proteinuria were uncommon. Hyperosmolar coma, polyuria nocturia and ketoacidosis were often absent or mild despite severe hyperglycemia. It was suggested that low blood pressure secondary to hypovolemia may protect against the development of vascular complications.

In a symposium held recently (1986) on diabetes mellitus in Saudi Arabia 10 of the 26 presentations were based on research work conducted in Saudi Arabia. Only one study was community based whereas the rest were carried out in hospitals. Only one study was published.[20] The following are some of the highlights of these studies.[21]

A study of 17,000 male and female Saudis in both urban and rural areas (Fatani et al.) showed relatively high prevalence rates of 4.95% in urban and 4.3% in rural communities. It was suggested that the rapid socioeconomic changes in the country over the last 20 years must have contributed to the high prevalence rates.

During a 5-year period (1981-1985) the records of 2,490 diabetic patients were reviewed at Riyadh Central Hospital (Hagaroo et al.). The ratio of NIDDM to IDDM was 4 to 1. A special tropical type "ketosis-resistant insulin type" was encountered in 44% of the IDDM patients (8% of all diabetics). These patients, despite insulin withdrawal for days or months, or even under stressful situation, did not develop ketoacidosis. Neurovascular microangiopathic complications were frequent in all groups. The overall compliance of patients with follow-up was poor.

Retinopathy was relatively common (24%) in 256 Saudi diabetic patients studied in King Abdul Aziz University Hospital, Riyadh.[21]

Three studies were concerned with diabetes among pregnant women. The results indicated that gestational diabetes is common among Saudi women.[21] It occurred in 1-5% of the studied women.[21] Infants of diabetic mothers were relatively larger than their expected weight. Congenital abnormalities were found only in the insulin dependent population; neither maternity deaths nor complications occurred.[21]

A study of 200 diabetic patients[21] indicated that both being overweight and a family history diabetes were strong predisposing factors. Nearly half (48%) of the newly diagnosed diabetics had complications mainly hypertension and neuropathy. Adult diabetics was mainly type 2, with only 10% of patients with low C-peptide levels. Another study in progress[21] suggested that diabetic Muslims can observe fasting in Ramadan provided that proper attention is paid to the control of the blood glucose.

At present, the staff of the Faculty of Medicine at the King Faisal University of Dammam have started a project to assess the problem of diabetes among the University hospital patients (personal communication).

WHICH WAY FORWARD?

Data on diabetes mellitus are still scarce in Saudi Arabia. The general impression from the limited literature available is that it is an emerging problem in Saudi Arabia particularly in urban societies. An increasing prevalence of the disorder could be related to the changes in social life and dietary pattern as a result of the rapid economic growth. People are resorting to foods rich in carbohydrates and fat and leading sedentary lives.

Because of the scarcity of data the epidemiology of the disease is not yet fully understood. Many questions regarding the magnitude of the problem, its distribution, contributing factors, pathogenesis and criteria for diagnosis still need to be answered.

Most of the studies carried out so far have been hospital-based dealing with small unrepresentative samples. There is an urgent need for collective efforts from researchers in universities and health service organizations to conduct more comprehensive and coordinated research work.

For proper control, programs of health education, early diagnosis and early treatment should always be emphasized. Health education should emphasize the importance of physical exercise, balanced diets, avoidance of being overweight, excessive worries and intermarriage, within diabetic families. Modifying the lifestyle of the people is probably the biggest challenge.

REFERENCES

1. **Cahill GF Jr.** Current concepts of diabetes. In: Marble A, Krall LP, Bradley RF, *et al.* eds. *Joslin's diabetes mellitus,* 12th edn. Philadelphia: Lea & Febiger, 1985; 1-11.
2. **Papper S.** Internal medicine. In: Frohlich ED ed. *Rypins' medical licensure examinations,* Philadelphia: JB Lipincott, 1981; 728-729.
3. **Berkow R,** ed. Diabetes mellitus. In: *Merk manual of diagnosis and therapy.* 14th edn. Rahway, New Jersey, USA: Merk & Co. Inc., 1982; 1037-1052.
4. **Scrimshow NS, Wray JD.** Nutrition and preventive medicine. In: Last JM, ed. *Maxcy-Rosenau public health and preventive medicine,* 11th edn. New York: Appleton-Century-Crofts, 1980; 1469-1503.
5. **Krolewski AS, Warram JH.** In: Marble A, Krall LP, Bradley RF, *et al.,* eds. *Joslin's diabetes mellitus,* 12th edn. Philadelphia: Lea & Febiger, 1985; 12-42.
6. **WHO Expert Committee on Diabetes Mellitus.** Technical Report Series 646. Geneva, World Health Organization 1980.
7. **Zimmet P.** Type 2 (noninsulin dependent) Diabetes. An epidemiologic overview. *Daibetologia* 1982; 22: 399-411.
8. **Neel JV.** Diabetes mellitus. A "Thrifty" genotype rendered detrimental by progress. *Am J Hum Genet* 1962; 14: 353-362.

9. **Bell JL, Chang P.** Glycosuria and diabetes mellitus in Saudi Arabia. *Saudi Med J* 1982; 3: 284-290.

10. **Bacchus RA, Bell JL, Madkour M. Kilshaw B.** The prevalence of diabetes mellitus in male Saudi Arabs. Diabetologia 1982; 23: 330-332.

11. **Bell JL, Bacchus RA, Madkour MM, Kilshaw BH.** The prevalence of diabetes mellitus in male and female Saudi Arabs. In: Bejaj JS *et al.* eds. *Diabetes mellitus in developing countries.* New Delhi Interprint 1984; 35-38.

12. **Bell JL, Bacchus RA.** Glucose tolerance in Saudi Arabs in relation to the criteria of the World Health Organization. *Saudi Med J* 1984; 5: 61-64.

13. **Bacchus R, Bell J.** Diabetes in Saudi Arabia. Hospimedica 1985; 9: 6-11.

14. **Kassimi MA, Khan MA.** Maturity onset diabetes of youth in Saudi patients: Is it a common problem? *Saudi Med J* 1981; 2: 146-148.

15. **Mathew PM, Hamdan JA.** *Presenting features and prevalence of juvenile diabetes mellitus in Saudi Arab children,* Aramco, Dhahran, Saudi Arabia: Pediat Service Division, 1982: 7 pp.

16. **Kyllo CJ, Nuttall FQ.** Prevalence of diabetes mellitus in school-age children in Minnesota. *Diabetes* 1978; 27: 57-60.

17. **Sterkey G, Holmgren G, Gustavson KH,** *et al.* The incidence of diabetes in Swedish children, 1970-1975. *Acta Pediat Scand* 1978; 67: 139-143.

18. **Joner G, Sovik O.** Incidence, age at onset and seasonal variation of diabetes mellitus in Norwegian children, 1973-1977. *Acta Pediat Scand* 1981; 70: 329-335.

19. **Lestradet H, Besse J.** Prevalence and incidence of diabetes mellitus in children and adolescents. *Acta Pediat Belg* 1977; 30: 123-124.

20. **Kingston M, Skoog WC.** Diabetes in Saudi Arabia. *Saudi Med J* 1986; 7: 130-142.

21. **bstracts.** *Symposium on diabetes mellitus in Saudi Arabia* held on 4-5 May 1986 at Medical City King Fahd National Guard Hospital, Riyadh. The Joint Board of Postgraduate Medical Education, King Saud University, Riyadh. 1986: 34 pp. (Abstracts).

DISORDERS OF HEMOGLOBIN SYNTHESIS

INTRODUCTION

Common red cell disorders include hemoglobinopathies, thalassemias and enzymopathies. Hemoglobinopathies result from structural defects in the hemoglobin molecule; the most common result from the presence of hemoglobin S.

Sickle cell disease (SCD) was first reported in 1910 as a chronic, hemolytic molecular disease that is genetically transmitted as an autosomal recessive disorder.[1, 2] Homozygotes for the abnormal gene suffer from sickle cell anemia while the heterozygous state is asymptomatic. The deoxygenation of hemoglobin causes a transition of the red cell from the normal to a sickle shape, thereby increasing its fragility, decreasing its survival rate, and subsequently causing hemolysis.

The highest incidence of the sickle-cell trait occurs in the eastern part of Africa where about 40% of the members of certain tribes are affected. In the USA overall prevalence among the Black population is 9%.

The clinical course of SCD is characterized by a steady state of chronic hemolysis, interrupted by "crises" which occur more commonly in early life and become less frequent during adulthood. There is a tendency towards vascular occlusion and a susceptibility to infection.

The thalassemia syndrome is due to a decreased rate of synthesis of one of the polypeptides of hemoglobin, thereby affecting the a/β chain rates. β-thalassemia is found in a broad belt extending from the Mediterranean basin through the Middle East to the Far East.[3] In homozygous β-thalassemia (Cooley's anemia, or thalassemia major) there is a considerable increase in the amount of fetal hemoglobin (HF) and the main effects are those of a very severe hemolytic anemia.

a-Thalassemia is especially common in South East Asia. In the homozygous state there is a complete inability to produce a chains, and the major component of Hb-Bart's (an abnormal form of fetal hemoglobin) is present. a-thalassemia major is incompatible with life, but a-thalassemia minor, found in individuals who are heterozygotes for the a-thalassemia gene, is symptomless.

There are several variants of glucose-6-phosphate dehydrogenase (G-6-PD) deficiency which produce different clinical pictures ranging from non-spherocytic hemolytic anemia to asymptomatic carriers. Glucose-6-phosphate dehydrogenase was first noted in Black Americans. It is also found in many Mediterranean and Far Eastern people in whom the clinical effects are more severe. Oxidant drugs like sulfones and sulfonamides, are liable to induce hemolysis. The acute hemolytic anemia called favism that occasionally occurs after ingestion of fava beans (*Vicia faba*) is seen in Mediterranean groups.

A combination of different hemoglobinophathies is quite common but none of these conditions is as severe as sickle cell anemia or thalassemia major.

HISTORICAL BACKGROUND

SICKLE CELL DISEASE

Anemia is a common health problem in the Arabian Peninsula and is caused by a variety of environmental factors and genetic abnormalities.[4] Until the mid-1950s not a single case of Sickle cell disease (SCD) had been diagnosed in Saudi Arabia. One factor which served to obscure the presence of SCD was holoendemic falciparum and vivax malaria which affected several oasis populations.[5]

A patient with anemia and splenomegaly was generally regarded as having malaria, even when parasites could not be demonstrated in blood films. Patients with jaundice and abdominal pain were often diagnosed as cases of viral hepatitis.[6] The discovery of the presence of the sickle cell gene, first in the Eastern Province, made physicians and scientists aware of the possible contribution of this genetic disorder to the overall picture of anemia. In 1967, the first case of thalassemia was also reported from the Eastern Province.[7]

Since Aramco (Arabian American Oil Company) operates in the Eastern Province and a high percentage of its employees come from the same area, an extensive research program was carried out there. Between 1955 and 1957 Marajian et al.[8] and Lehmann et al.[9] examined adult male Saudi Arabs in the Eastern Province for the presence of sickle cell hemoglobin. The frequency of sickling (AS) was 25.1% among the Shiite population (a sect of Islam), 10.2% among Sunnite townspeople (a majority sect of Islam), 1% among settled populations coming from other provinces, and none at all among Bedouins. The Shiite population exhibits the highest frequency of the sickle cell trait of any population in the Middle East.[6]

Between 1973 and 1975, a survey was carried out on 88,084 adult Saudi males, all residents of the Eastern Province.[10] The survey revealed 872 cases with the sickle cell trait (AS) and 51 with SCD. The majority of the group with SCD showed mild-to-moderate anemia. A mild course for sickle cell disease and thalassemias was also observed in several other studies.[4, 6, 11]

The clinical course was believed to be significantly modified as a result of both the high HbF and the interaction of the sickle gene with other genetic abnormalities such as the thalassemias and G-6-PD deficiency. Saudi patients, in general, present with unexplained anemia, recurrent bone and/or joint pain, occasionally with abdominal or back pain, and at times with illnesses unrelated to SCD. Patients do not exhibit the asthenic, eunuchoid habitus or ulcerations of the lower extremities typical of homozygous SCD among Americans of African origin. The most consistent physical abnormality is the presence of splenomegaly and hepatomegaly. Complications directly attributable to SCD are unusual.[6]

In 1976, El-Hazmi and Lehmann [12] reported a new structurally abnormal hemoglobin variant, Hb Riyadh.

Perrine et al.[13] reported the results of their study of 270 Saudi children with homozygous sickle cell anemia, 74% presented with anemia.

Compared with American or Jamaican Blacks, serious complications occurred only 6-25% as frequently in the Saudis; leg ulcers did not occur at all; mortality under 15 years of age was 10% as great; mean levels of blood hemoglobin were higher (10g/dl compared to 7.9 g/dl), and reticulocyte count was lower (5% compared to 6%).

Pembrey et al.[14] measured fetal hemoglobin (HbF) levels in 137 normal (AA) subjects, 109 with the sickle cell trait (AS) and 237 with sickle cell anemia (SS) in the population of the Eastern Province. In addition, he estimated the proportion of F cells in 71 (AA), 51 (AS) and 34 (SS) subjects. The mean HbF% (and the range of F cells %) were: (AA) 0.77 (0.3-18), (AS) 1.38 (2.3-43) and (SS) 25.56 (33-98). Whilst the (AA) and (AS) subjects did not differ from comparable groups of American Blacks, both the HbF% and F cells % in (SS) subjects were much higher than in American Blacks.

Pembrey et al.[15] found that remarkably high levels of HbF in the Eastern Province of Saudi Arabia were not restricted to individuals with sickle cell anemia but also occurred in compound heterozygotes for the sickle cell and β-thalassemia genes.

Sickle cell disease in Saudi Arabia is associated with an unusually high level of fetal hemoglobin. Red cells containing more HbF have a greater chance of survival in the circulation. The HbF level showed an inverse correlation with the degree of hemolysis. This phenomenon is attributed to an interference by high HbF with the aggregation of HbS molecules, thus minimizing sickling.[16]

Hemoglobin S and HbF both provide resistance against *Plasmodium falciparum*.[17,18] HbS appears to impair the growth of the malaria parasite by the formation of molecular aggregates, the formation of which are also enhanced by the lowering of the oxygen partial pressure and the intracellular pH by the parasite.[19]

Mortality due to malaria selectively removes the genetically normal individuals.[18] This leads to an increased frequency in the population of the allele controlling hemoglobin S. This selective mechanism, in addition to consanguinity, may add to the increase of the sickle cell gene frequency over the years in malarious environments.

Saudi subjects with homozygous sickle cell disease survive to adult life, and under these circumstances, the contribution to the gene pool from SS individuals is significant.

Sickle cell disease has become a major health problem of increasing importance because of the virtual disappearance of so many infectious, parasitic, and nutritional disorders which previously affected the Saudi population.[6]

The researches of Gelpi[20] led to the hypothesis that the sickle cell gene appeared as an isolated mutation in equatorial Africa and that its current distribution in Europe and Asia represents the combined effects of major population movements, the changing epidemiology of *P. falciparum* malaria, interaction of hemoglobin S with the thalassemias and G-6-PD deficiency, and, possibly, the capacity of certain individuals with sickle cell disease to generate large amounts of fetal hemoglobin.

THALASSEMIA

Where the sickle cell gene is common, thalassemias co-exist at a relatively higher frequency than in other regions.[4]

The oasis populations of Eastern Saudi Arabia have one of the highest recorded gene frequencies for a-thalassemia.[21]

The presence of increased amounts of HbBart's (a_4) in the neonatal period is a sensitive indicator of the a-thalassemia gene.[22] Pembrey et al.[23] in 1975 examined the hemoglobin pattern of 345 Shiite Saudi Arab cord bloods. HbBart's was found in 52% of the cases, the highest incidence of this variant yet recorded and an indication of the presence of a high frequency of a-thalassemia.

Hemoglobin H (β_4) disease, the most important form of a-thalassemia, is a chronic hemolytic anemia found commonly in the Orient and Mediterranean. McNiel[24] was the first to describe hemoglobin H disease in the Saudi population in 1973. He recognized that its genetic transmission did not follow the pattern observed commonly in Orientals.

A study of 11 families with a-thalassemia in the Qatif oasis indicated that McNiel's suggestion was correct.[25] There are two common molecular forms of a-thalassemia, a deletion (-a) determinant and a non-deletion (aa+) determinant, which interact to produce a series of closely overlapping phenotypes. The most severe hemoglobin H disease results from the homozygous state of the non-deletion determinant, a pattern of inheritance not previously recognized for this condition.

The sickle cell β-thalassemia, with virtually no production of hemoglobin A, may be the most frequent type of SCD encountered among Saudi adults.[6] About 10% of Saudi subjects with sickle cell disease have β-thalassemia.[26]

GLUCOSE-6-PHOSEPHTE DEHYDROGENASE (G-6-PD) DEFICIENCY

In 1965, Gelpi[27] conducted a survey of G-6-PD deficiency among 1296 Saudi subjects. Of randomly selected subjects 13% of males and 24% of females were found to be G-6-PD deficient; G-6-PD deficiency showed a low frequency in Bedouin tribes and a rather higher frequency in tribes of African origin.[28]

Gelpi[29] found a significant association between hemoglobin S and G-6-PD deficiency in the Eastern Province. Almost 60% of male subjects with the sickle cell trait have been observed to have G-6-PD deficiency.[30, 31] This association has not been observed in other populations of Asia or Africa with the exception of Ghana.[32] A plausible explanation for the association is that the sickle cell trait and G-6-PD deficiency together provide a greater selective advantage than either red cell defect alone.

El-Hazmi and Warsy[33] found that among the Saudi HbS homozygotes the hematological parameters in the presence of G-6-PD deficiency are improved and so are the clinical manifestations. The prevalences of anemia, splenomegaly, and jaundice are lower in the G-6-PD deficient HbS homozygotes. The possibility is that sickle cell anemia modifies the phenotypic expression of G-6-PD deficiency, and G-6-PD deficiency may in some way mitigate full expression of homozygous SCD.[32]

The high frequency of G-6-PD deficiency among subjects with the sickling trait supports the hypothesis that G-6-PD deficiency provides a qualitatively similar selective advantage against falciparum malaria to that enjoyed by those subjects with the sickling trait.[34] However, falciparum malaria does not appear to be the only significant factor determining marked regional differences in the incidence of G-6-PD. This genetic marker is essentially confined to the Shiite Moslem population. The Sunni population, regardless of its proximity to areas of endemic falciparum malaria, has a low incidence of G-6-PD deficiency.

THE PRESENT SITUATION: THE 1980S

The sickle cell gene is unevenly distributed in the Arabian Peninsula. It is more frequently encountered in agricultural regions where malaria used to be endemic. There are three main pockets for the sickling gene where the thalassemias and G-6-PD deficiency are also frequently encountered.[35] These are the Qatif and Al-Hasa oases (Eastern Province),

Khaiber (North West) and Tehamat-Aseer (South West). All these are agricultural areas where malaria was, or still is endemic.

Perrine et al.[11] screened 2,341 infants from the Eastern Province. Of these, 78% were normal, 20% had the sickle cell trait, 1.58% had homozygous sickle cell anemia and 0.25% had sickle-β_0 thalassemia. On follow-up from birth (or from 3 months) for a mean of 3.5 years there was more morbidity and mortality than in matched Saudi Arab controls, but these rates were lower than for affected Black infants in the USA or Jamaica. The fetal hemoglobin level was high (32%) at 4-5 years. Half of a subsample of 23 cases had evidence of co-existent a-thalassemia.

The pregnancy complications were studied in 601 pregnant Saudi females with sickle cell anemia, the sickle cell trait, and with no HbS in the Eastern Province.[36] No maternal death was recorded in any of the three groups studied. The incidences of abortion, premature deliveries and perinatal mortality were higher in pregnant females with HbS-S than in the other two groups. An increased incidence of pre-eclamptic toxemia, and infectious complications was also noted in pregnant women with sickle cell anemia. The mean birth weight for infants born to mothers with HbS-S was 372 gm less than those born to sickle-negative mothers. The pregnancy experiences of women with the sickle cell trait were not different from those in whom red cells do not sickle.

The function of the spleen was assessed in 20 Eastern Province Saudis with sickle cell anemia.[37] Four of the 20 patients had a definitely reduced function of the spleen, and these patients tended to have lower fetal hemoglobin levels and a more severe clinical history. By comparison with previous studies on American Blacks with sickle cell anemia the spleen appears to function better and for a longer time in the majority of Saudis with SCD. It has been suggested that the high fetal hemoglobin level in Saudis is the main determinant of the less severe hematological picture.

El-Hazmi[4] conducted a survey in different villages in Tehamat-Aseer. The sickle cell hemoglobin was detected in about 8-27% of the population and the prevalence of G-6-PD deficiency ranged between 8-15%; a-thalassemia and β-thalassemia gene frequencies varied between 20-30% and 10-15%, respectively.

In a study of the frequency of HbS, thalassemia and G-6-PD deficiency genes in the North Western Province, the results showed major interregional differences.[38] Khaiber, a traditionally agricultural area with a high incidence of malaria, a fairly closed community with very limited movement of population, and a high rate of cousin intermarriage, has the highest gene frequency for HbS and G-6-PD deficiency and a fairly high frequency of a and β-thalassemia. The mild nature of the genetic diseases agree with the findings in other areas of the Kingdom.

The malaria-free regions of Saudi Arabia are fundamentally free from the mutant genes. A hematological study of 436 pregnant women in Khamis Mishait, Asir (22,300 m altitude and a malaria-free area), revealed no SCD or thalassemia.[39] Another study of 257 pre-school children in Tamnia villages, Asir, revealed no SCD, one case of HbH and some cases of microcytic hypochromic anemia, a possible indication of a-thalassemia.[40]

Bayoumi et al.[28] studied abnormal hemoglobins and G-6-PD deficiencies in 638 subjects (all Sunni Moslems) from six tribes in Western Saudi Arabia including two tribes of African origin. No sickling or a very low rate of sickling was found in the indigenous Arab tribes. In contrast, the frequency of HbS in the two tribes of African origin was relatively high. Lehmann et al.[41] also found no sicklers among Bedouins. The authors supported Gelpi's theory[20] that the origin of HbS was in Africa.

Besides inherited factors such as high HbF, thalassemia, and G-6-PD deficiency which might affect the severity of SCD, some acquired anemias, such as iron deficiency anemia, may contribute to the mild clinical presentation of the sickle cell disease.[42] It was found that the red cells do not sickle *in vitro* until the hemoglobin concentration in the blood is raised to 10% with iron supplementation.[43] Wishner[44] also observed that at a low hemoglobin concentration, the deoxygenated HbS has the same structure as HbA.

In 1980, the first case of HbO Arab was reported in Saudi Arabia.[45] The patient was a Saudi female doubly heterozygous for HbO Arab and thalassemia. It has been suggested that the discovery of HbO Arab in Saudi Arabia may indicate that the recent patients with HbO detected in the East of the country using paper electrophoresis as the only means of identification[46] may in fact have been patients with HbO Arab.

CONTROL

The frequency of the sickle cell trait is the result of two opposing processes of natural selection, the deaths of homozygotes from sickle cell anemia and the deaths of normals from malaria. Its frequency in a population is related to the recent malarial history of that population.

Sickle cell anemia has no definitive cure. However, better living conditions, balanced nutrition and general medical care usually result in better prognoses. Theoretically, one can change the DNA, transplant bone marrow, increase fetal hemoglobin synthesis, and provide conditions or compounds which can increase erythrocyte oxygen affinity, decrease deoxyhemoglobin S polymerization and decrease sickle cell membrane damage[47, 48]

The use of amino acids and short peptides, the feasibility of designing molecules that will react with amino acids in specific sites on the hemoglobin molecule, the extracorporeal treatment of blood with anti-sickling agents and the work at "gene" level are just some of the current lines of research.[49]

Early screening is recommended for infants at risk for SCD and comprehensive care should be given even if the infant has the less severe type of hemoglobinopathies. Intermarriage between relatives (consanguinity) should not be encouraged.

REFERENCES

1. **Neel JV.** The inheritance of sickle cell anemia, *Science* 1949; 110: 64-66.

2. **Pauling L, Itano HA, Singer SJ, Well IC.** Sickle cell anemia, a molecular disease, *Science* 1949; 110: 543-548.

3. **Walters JH.** The tropical anemias. In: Wilcocks and Manson-Bahr, eds. *Mansons' tropical disease.* London: Bailliere Tindall, 1972: 21-37.

4. **El-Hazmi MAF.** The red cell genetics and environmental interactions - a Tehamat-Aseer profile. *Saudi Med J* 1985; 6: 101-112.

5. **Daggy RH.** Malaria in oases of Eastern Saudi Arabia. II, *Am J Trop Med Hyg* 1959; 8: 223-291.

6. **Gelpi AP.** Sickle cell disease in Saudi Arabia. *Acta Haematol* 1970; 43: 89-99.

7. **McNiel JR.** Family studies of thalassemia in Arabia. *Am J Hum Genet* 1967; 19: 100-111.

8. **Marajian G, Ikin EW, Mourant AE, Lehmann H.** The blood groups and haemoglobins of the Saudi Arabians. *Hum Biol* 1966; 38: 394-420.

9. **Lehmann H, Marajian G, Mourant AE.** Distribution of sickle cell haemoglobin in Saudi Arabia. *Nature* 1963; 198: 492-493.

10. **Gelpi AP.** Benign sickle cell disease in Saudi Arabia: survival estimate and population dynamics. *Clin Genet* 1979; 15: 307-310.

11. **Perrine RP, John P, Pembrey M, Perrine S.** Sickle cell disease in Saudi Arabs in early childhood. *Arch Dis Child* 1981; 56: 187-192.

12. **El-Hazmi MAF, Lehmann H.** Haemoglobin Riyadh - A2B2(120(GH3) Lys-Asn). A new variant found in association with a-thalassemia: and iron deficiency. *Haemoglobin* 1976; 1: 59-74.

13. **Perrine RP, Pembrey ME, John P, Perrine S, Shoup F.** Natural history of sickle cell anaemia in Saudi Arabia. *Ann Int Med* 1978; 88: 1-6.

14. **Pembrey ME, Wood WG, Weatherall DJ, Perrine RP.** Foetal hemoglobin production and the sickle gene in the oases of Eastern Saudi Arabia. *Br J Haematol* 1978; 40: 415-429.

15. **Pembrey ME, Perrine RP, Wood WG, Weatherall DJ.** Sickle-β-thalassemia in Eastern Saudi Arabia. *Am J Hum Genet* 1980; 32: 26-41.

16. **Bertles JF, Rabinovitz R, Dobler J.** Haemoglobin interaction; modification of solid phase composition in the sickling phenomenon. *Science* 1970; 169: 375-378.

17. **Pasvol G, Weatherall DJ, Wilson RJM.** Effects of feotal haemoglobin on susceptibility of red cells to plasmodium falciparum. *Nature* 1977; 270: 171-173.

18. **Pasvol G. Weatherall DJ, Wilson RJM.** Cellular mechanism for the protective effect of haemoglobin S against P. falciparum malaria. *Nature* 1978; 247: 701-703.

19. **Roth EF, Friedman M, Ueda Y, Tellez I, Trager W, Nagel RL.** Sickling rates of human AS red cells infected in vitro with Plasmodium falciparum malaria. *Science* 1978; 202: 650-652.

20. Gelpi AP. Migrant populations and the diffusion of the sickle-cell gene. *Ann Int Med* 1973; 79: 258-264.

21. **Weatherall DJ, Clegg JB.** *The thalassemia syndromes.* 2d ed. Oxford: Blackwell, 1972.

22. **Weatherall DJ.** Abnormal haemoglobins in the neonatal period and their relationship to thalassemia. _Br J Haematol_ 1963; 9: 265.

23. **Pembrey ME, Weatherall DJ, Clegg JB, Bunch C, Perrine RP.** Haemoglobin Bart's in Saudi Arabia. _Br J Haematol_ 1975; 29: 221-234.

24. McNiel JR. Family studies of alpha-thalassemia and hemoglobin H disease in Eastern Saudi Arabia. _J Med Assoc Thai_ 1971; 54: 153-166.

25. **Pressley L, Higgs DR, Clegg JB, Perrine RP, Pembrey ME, Weatherall DJ.** A new genetic basis for hemoglobin-H disease. _New Engl J Med_ 1980; 3: 1383-1388.

26. **Perrine RP, Pembrey ME, John P, Perrine S, Shoup F.** Natural history of sickle cell anemia in Saudi Arabia. _Ann Int Med_ 1978; 88: 1-6.

27. **Gelpi AP.** Glucose-6-phosphate dehydrogenase deficiency in Saudi Arabia. _Blood_ 1965; 25: 486-493.

28. **Bayoumi RA, Omer A, Samuel APW, Saha N, Sebai ZA, Sabaa HMA.** Haemoglobin and erythrocytic glucose-6-phosphate dehydrogenase variants among selected tribes in Western Saudi Arabia. _Trop Geog Med_ 1979; 31: 245-252.

29. **Gelpi AP, King MC.** New data on glucose-6-phosphate dehydrogenase deficiency in Saudi Arabia. _Hum Hered_ 1977; 27: 285-291.

30. **Gelpi AP.** Glucose-6-phosphate dehydrogenase deficiency, the sickling trait, and malaria in Saudi Arab children. _J Pediat_ 1967; 71: 138-146.

31. **Gelpi AP.** Glucose-6-phosphate dehydrogenase deficiency in Saudi Arabia. _Bull WHO_ 1967; 37: 539-546.

32. **Lewis RA, Hathorn M.** Correlation of S hemoglobin with glucose-6-phosphate dehydrogenase deficiency and its significance. _Blood_ 1965; 26: 176-180.

33. **El-Hazmi MAF, Warsy AS.** Aspects of sickle cell gene in Saudi Arabia - interaction with glucose-6-phosphate dehydrogenase deficiency. _Hum Genet_ 1984; 68: 320-323.

34. **Gelpi AP.** Glucose-6-phosphate dehydrogenase deficiency: the sickling trait, and malaria in Saudi Arab children. _J Pediat_ 1967; 71: 138-146.

35. **El-Hazmi MAF.** Haemoglobin disorders: a pattern for thalassaemia and haemoglobinopathies in Arabia. *Acta Haematol* 1982; 68: 43-51.

36. **Kandil OF, Saleh AA, Khater RA, Mohammed AM, Hindawy DS.** The course and outcome of pregnancy in Saudi females with sickle cell anaemia and sickle cell trait. In: *Proceedings of the 7th Saudi Medical Meeting.* Dammam: King Faisal University, 1982: 360-365.

37. **Al-Awamy B, Pearson HA, Wilson WA, Naeem MA.** Function of the spleen in Saudi patients with sickle cell anaemia. In: *Proceedings of the 7th Saudi Medical Meeting.* Dammam: King Faisal University, 1982: 439-445.

38. **El-Hazmi MAF.** Incidence and frequency of haemoglobinopathies and thalassaemia in the North-West sector of Arabia. *Saudi Med J* 1985; 6: 149-162.

39. **Hartley DRW.** One thousand obstetric deliveries in the Asir Province, Kingdom of Saudi Arabia: a review. *Saudi Med J* 1980; 1: 187-196.

40. **El-Hazmi MAF, Sebai ZA.** Laboratory tests profile for pre-school children at Tamnia (Aseer Province). *Saudi Med J* 1981; 2: 198-202.

41. **Lehmann H. Maranijan G, Mourant AE.** Distribution of sickle-cell haemoglobin in Saudi Arabia. Nature, Lond 1963; 198-492.

42. **El-Hazmi MAF.** Human haemoglobin and haemoglobinopathies in the Arabian Peninsula - studies at the molecular level. In: *Proceedings of the 4th Saudi Medical Conference.* Dammam: King Faisal University, 1980; 317-324.

43. **Greenberg MS, Kass EH, Castle WB.** Studies in the destruction of red cells. XII. Factors influencing the role of S haemoglobin in the pathologic physiology of sickle-cell anemia and related disorders. *J Clin Invest* 1957; 36: 833-847.

44. **Wishner BC, Ward KB, Lattman EE, Love WE.** Crystal structure of sickle cell deoxyhaemoglobin at 5 A° resolution. *J Mol Biol* 1975; 98: 179-194.

45. **El-Hazmi MAF, Lehmann H.** Human haemoglobins and haemoglobinopathies in Arabia: Hb O Arab in Saudi Arabia. *Acta Haematol* 1980; 63: 268-273.

46. **Gelpi AP, King MC.** Screening for abnormal hemoglobins in the Middle East: new data on hemoglobin S and the presence

of hemoglobin C in Saudi Arabia. *Acta Haematol* 1976; 56: 334-337.

47. **Brewer GJ, Brewer LF, Prasad AS.** Suppression of irreversibly sickled erythrocytes by zinc therapy in sickle cell anemia. *J Lab Clin Med* 1977; 90: 549-554.

48. **Brewer GJ, Bereza U.** Membrane therapy of sickle cell anemia with zinc and other drugs. In: Fried W, ed. *Comparative clinical aspects of sickle cell disease.* New York, Elsevier/North Holland, 1982: 175-187.

49. **Warsy AS, El-Hazmi MAF, Bahakim HM.** Molecular therapy of sickle cell anaemia - the state of the art. *Saudi Med J* 1985; 6: 257-263.

CANCERS

INTRODUCTION

Neoplastic diseases are generally assumed to be related to an uncontrolled growth of cells with an invasion of the adjacent normal tissues and a spread to other parts of the body. They may arise in any part of the body and involve any type of cells. A tumor, in this state of continued growth at the expense of the host has been defined as an autonomous parasite. In 1975 cancer was the second most common cause of death in the USA.

The majority of cancers have no apparent cause. However, a variety of environmental factors (chemical, physical and biological) have been implicated as causal agents for different forms of cancer. The possible interaction between genetic and environmental factors as well as the immunological concepts are under detailed investigation. The most successful approach to the control of cancer lies in its prevention; primary prevention by avoiding carcinogenic agents and secondary prevention by early detection and treatment.

Table 1. Main Studies Published on Cancer in Saudi Arabia.

First Author	Year of Publication	Ref. No.	Topic	Location	No. of Patients
Taylor	1963	(2)	General	Aramco	264
Gelpi	1970	(5)	Lymphoma	Aramco	43
Perrine	1975	(4)	General	Aramco	-
Sayigh	1977	(55)	Skin	CLR	3,251
El-Faraidi	1979	(67)	Esophagus	RKH	-
Stirling	1979	(6,7)	General	CLJ	1,000
Atiyeh	1980	(30)	Liver	KFSH	54
Jamjoom	1980	(41)	Breast	KAUH	22
Macaron	1980	(40)	Thyroid	KFSH	35
Monib	1980	(29)	GI and liver	KFH	67
Sabbah	1980	(58)	Retinoblastoma	KFSH	20
Shobokshi	1980	(27)	GIT	KAUH	551

Main Author	Year of Publication	Ref. No.	Topic	Location	No. of Patients
Stirling	1981	(38)	Mouth	KAUH	154
Amer	1982	(15)	General	KFSH	1,000
Al-Karawi	1982	(26)	Esophagus	RKH	1,550
Bin Ahmed	1982	(8)	Lymphoma	KFSH	100
El-Akkad	1982	(68)	Control	KFSH	-
Mughal	1982	(56)	Melanoma	KFSH	22
Mee	1982	(47)	Bladder	-	-
El-Akkad	1983	(14)	General	KFSH	1,696
Hannan	1984	(53)	Skin	KFSH	1,296
Hanash	1984	(49)	Bladder	KFSH	-
Koriech	1984	(16)	General	RKH	297
Amer	1985	(28)	Esophagus	KFSH	98
Amer	1985	(39)	Oral	KFSH	68
Aur	1985	(17)	Leukemia	KFSH	91
Bedikian	1985	(62-64)	Behavior	KFSH	100
El-Akkad	1986	(1)	General	KFSH	7,251

ARAMCO	- Aramco Hospital, Dhahran
CLJ	- Central Laboratory, Jeddah
CLR	- Central Laboratory, Riyadh
KFSH	- King Faisal Specialist Hospital, Riyadh
KAUH	- King Abdul Aziz University Hospital, Jeddah
RKH	- Riyadh Al-Kharj Hospital, Riyadh
KFH	- King Faisal Hospital, Taif

Several studies on cancer have been undertaken in Saudi Arabia, mostly of an epidemiological nature, to define the magnitude of the problem. Table 1 lists *several* according to the main author, year of publication, nature of study, location and number of patients. All the studies were hospital based, thus the results are not representative of a region or the country as a whole. Patients were by and large Saudis with a small minority of non-Saudis included.

In the absence of a national survey or national cancer registration these studies are the only source of information on cancer to date.

A comparison of prevalence or incidence between Saudi Arabia and other countries is quite difficult because of a lack of information on the base population and differences in age distribution. Even so, these studies still illustrate certain features of cancer in Saudi Arabia.

A recent study by El Akkad et al. (1986)[1] which covered 7,251 new cases of cancer seen over a 6-year period (1979-1984) at the King Faisal Specialist Hospital and Research Center in Riyadh (the main referral hospital for cancer patients in Saudi Arabia) shows the crude relative frequencies of cancer at various primary sites according to rank order and sex (Table 2).

The most prevailing cancers among males are non-Hodgkin's lymphomas, and cancer of the esophagus, lung, liver and stomach; whereas among females it is breast cancer, non-Hodgkin's lymphomas, and cancer of the thyroid, esophagus and cervix. When these results are compared with those of Taylor[2], who, 25 years previously, published the first paper on cancer in Saudi Arabia based on Aramco (Arabian-American Oil Company) Hospital statistics, the difference in the size of the problem and the rank order of the 14 top cancers can be seen (Table 3). At that time Aramco Hospital was almost the only referral hospital for cancer patients in Saudi Arabia.

Zohair A. Sebai

In Taylor's study (1950-1961) the male to female ratio was 2.7 to 1 and the peak incidence occurred in the age group of 41-50 years for males and 21-40 years for females. By 1984 the peak incidence increased by about 20 years for each sex (60-64 years for males and 50-54 years for females) and the sex ratio became 1.3 to 1.

Table 2. Crude Relative Frequency(CRF) and Rank Order of 7,251 Cancer Patients Seen at KFSH in Riyadh (1979-1984).

	Both Sexes		Males		Females	
Rank		CRF		CRF		CRF
Order	Description	%	Description	%	Description	%
1	Non-Hodgkin's lymphomas	10.3	Non-Hodgkin's lymphomas	12	Breast	17.2
2	Breast	7.6	Esophagus	6	Non-Hodgkin's lymphoma	7.9
3	Esophagus	5.6	Lung	5.8	Thyroid	5.6
4	Lung	4.3	Liver	5	Esophagus	4.9
5	Oral cavity	4.3	Stomach	5	Cervix	4.6
6	Lymphoid leukemia	3.8	Nasopharynx	4.7	Ovary	4.5
7	Stomach	3.8	Hodgkins	4.6	Oral cavity	4.4
8	Thyroid	3.7	Lymphoid leukemia	4.5	Myeloid leukemia	3.7
9	Nasopharynx	3.6	Oral cavity	4.1	Uterus	3
10	Hodgkins	3.6	CNS	3.9	CNS	2.9
11	Liver	3.5	Skin	3.8	Lymphoid leukemia	2.9
12	Myeloid leukemia	3.5	Bladder	3.7	Stomach	2.7
13	CNS	3.5	Myeloid leukemia	3.3	Skin (non-melanoma)	2.5
14	Skin (non-melanoma)	3.2	Bone sarcoma	2.6	Nasopharynx	2.3

Table 3. Rank Order of Cancers Among Males in Two Studies.

	Taylor* 1950-1961	El-Akkad** 1979-1984
No. of Patients	264	7,251
Rank Order		
1.	Stomach	Non-Hodgkin's lymphomas
2.	Lymphosarcoma	Esophagus
3.	Leukemia	Lung
4.	Lymphoma	Liver
5.	Skin	Stomach
6.	Esophagus	Nasopharynx
7.	Liver	Hodgkins
8.	Myeloma	Lymphoid leukemia
9.	Reticulum cell sarcoma	Oral cavity
10.	Rectum	CNS
11.	Hodgkin's	Skin
12.	Lung	Bladder
13.	Head and neck	Myeloid leukemia
14.	Bladder	Bone sarcoma

*Ref. 2.   **Ref. 1.

N.B. If in Taylor's study lymphosarcoma, lymphoma and reticulum cell sarcoma were all classified together as non-Hogkin's lymphoma this would be the first ranking category.

The differences shown in this comparison may also be due to variations in location, lifespan of the people involved, methods of diagnosis, availability of health services, or improved public awareness.

Taylor in 1963 wrote:[2] "Saudi women are resistant to medical examination. They were particularly resistant when they had tumors of the breast or genitalia and when male doctors were involved in further diagnosis and treatment. As further evidence of the backward nature of this society,* husbands have something to say about this and frequently refuse further medical attention for their wives." Women in the 1980s apparently became more acceptant of medical examination and treatment.[1]

---

*   A lack of understanding of the culture (author)

The peak incidence of age in the two studies is still low for both sexes compared to that in Western societies. This could be due to a shorter life expectancy[3] or a higher incidence of lymphomas and leukemias which affect young age groups.

There are noticeable differences in the relative frequency of cancers between different regions in Saudi Arabia which reflect the diversity of the geography, climate, urbanization, availability of medical care, dietary pattern, educational level and lifestyle of the people in different parts of the Kingdom. In the following sections, the epidemiology of the predominant types of cancers in Saudi Arabia will be discussed in the light of the available literature.

LYMPHOMAS

Taylor (1963)[2] observed the predominant incidence of tumors of the hemic and lymphatic systems among Aramco Hospital patients. When counted together they totaled 70 cases in a series of 264 cases (26.5%); an unusually high incidence of cancer of these systems as judged by Western standards. Perrine (1975),[4] in his follow-up study of Aramco patients in 1975 found several changes from Taylor's findings but lymphomas and leukemias were still the most common cancers.

Gelpi (1970)[5] published his study of 43 patients with malignant lymphomas diagnosed over a 15-year period (1953-1967) in the Aramco Hospital in Dhahran. The majority of the cases (53%) were lymphosarcomas. Of the entire group, 42% presented with primary abdominal lymphomas and 79% had abdominal involvement as a major manifestation of lymphoma when first seen.

Stirling (1977),[6, 7] in his study conducted in Jeddah, found that malignant lymphoma comprised 15% of all malignant tumors. Of the lymphomas 33% presented as primary abdominal malignancies.

The 100 cases of non-Hodgkin's Lymphoma examined by Bin Ahmed & Sabbah (1982)[8] comprised 17% of all malignant tumors seen over 5 years in King Faisal Specialist Hospital, Riyadh. Of the total, 79% presented with the abdominal form whereas primary abdominal lymphoma in Western countries is uncommon.[9] Seventeen cases had Burkitt's lymphoma; nine of these were referred from the Southern Province where malaria is common.

There is evidence that lymphomas may be the most frequent type of malignancy encountered - not only in Saudi Arabia but also in other Middle Eastern countries. They comprise 17.5% of all malignant diseases in Jordan, Syria and Lebanon,[3] 15.7% in Egypt[10] and 14% in Aden.[11] Except for a few African countries, the Middle East shows the highest incidence of lymphomas in the world.[12, 13]

El-Akkad in two consecutive studies in the periods 1975-1978[14] and 1979-1984[1] found that lymphomas come at the top of the list among males and second to breast cancer among females (Table 2).

A high frequency of lymphomas was also reported in other studies conducted in Jeddah and Riyadh Hospitals.[15, 16] Aur *et al.* (1985)[17] published the preliminary results of a protocol devised for the treatment of children with acute lymphocytic leukemia, previously untreated in the Kingdom of Saudi Arabia.

The predominance of lymphomas in the Middle East suggests ethnic or geographical factors, and further studies on the subject are required.

CANCER OF THE ESOPHAGUS

There is a great variation around the world in the incidence of cancer of the esophagus.[18] The prevalence varies from 5/100,000 in Western populations[19] to over 100/100,000 in some areas in the USSR, Iran, China and South Africa.[20] Globally it has a patchy distribution. For example, within a small area in northern China the mortality rate ranges from 1.4/100,000 to 140/100,000.[21]

Studies in different parts of the world have associated cancer of the esophagus with a variety of factors including excessive alcohol consumption, heavy cigarette smoking, thermal injuries resulting from drinking very hot beverages, physical injuries caused by ingesting very coarse food, vitamin A deficiency, and the exposure to some potentially mitogenic trace elements such as beryllium, cadmium or lead.[9, 20, 22, 23, 24, 25,]

In Saudi Arabia there is a high occurrence of cancer of the esophagus.[6, 14, 15] In a recent study[1] it was found to rank third after lymphomas and breast cancer. The disease showed a patchy distribution. In a 4-year period (1980-1983), 4,761 cancer patients were treated in King Faisal Specialist Hospital in Riyadh, 98 of whom had esophageal cancer (5%).[28] Although only 4% of all cancer patients came from the Qasim region, 20% of the esophageal cancer patients came from the same region ($p < 0.05$).

When esophageal cancer patients referred from Qasim were compared with those referred from other locations, no statistical differences were noted between the two groups except for the type and source of drinking water.[28] Water analysis in Qasim confirmed the presence of traces of methane gas and a high concentration of metalliferous minerals such as silver, gold and copper which suggests the presence of other minerals and trace elements in the region. Water contamination from materials such as petroleum oils, polycyclic hydrocarbons or other trace elements may be the main reason for the higher frequency of cancer of the esophagus in Qasim.

Other features of interest in the same study[28] were that 14% of the patients had carcinoma in the upper esophagus, 34% in the middle third, and 52% in the lower third. A family history of cancer was found in only one patient; 22% of the patients were cachectic (less than 40 kg in weight), 35% had features of mild vitamin A deficiency; and most patients in this study drank more than 10 cups of extremely hot Arabic coffee per day. Obviously, further studies are needed to define the etiology of cancer of the esophagus in Saudi Arabia.

CANCER OF THE STOMACH

The frequency of stomach cancer in Saudi Arabia varied in different studies. Taylor, in the 1950s, found it the most common single type of tumor among Aramco patients.[2] Perrine[4] found a high incidence in the Eastern Province, where it ranked third in males and fourth in females. In the study conducted by El-Akkad[1] on King Faisal Specialist Hospital patients, the tumor ranked seventh of all tumors among both sexes, being fifth among males and twelfth among females. The highest frequency was among patients from the Central and Northern Provinces (5.8% of all tumors) and the lowest was among patients from Jeddah (2.8%). El-Akkad believed that the occurrence of the lowest rate in Jeddah was due to the impact of modernization. If this is true, the incidence of stomach cancer should decline in the future as it has in other parts of the world.

PRIMARY HEPATOCELLULAR CARCINOMA

Primary hepatocellular carcinoma (PHC), an uncommon disease in Europe and North America, has a high incidence in the developing world, especially in the Orient, South East Asia and Africa.

It is a rather common tumor in Saudi Arabia although it varies in frequency according to time and place. In various studies it ranked fourth[2,]

[4] and sixteenth[6] among other tumors. Factors influencing these variations need to be further investigated.

Monib,[29] in his study of 67 cases of patients with gastrointestinal carcinoma, found a high incidence of cancer of the liver (48%). Most patients came in an advanced condition and the mortality rate was 100%.

Korriech & Al Kuhaymi[16] found that gastrointestinal malignancies account for about one-fifth of all malignancies with a predominance of esophageal and liver cancers.

Atiyeh's study[30] of 54 cases of PHC has shed some light on the clinicopathological aspects of the disease. The majority of patients were between 60 and 70 years old. The male to female ratio was 10 to 1. The most common presenting symptoms were upper abdominal pain, dyspepsia, abdominal swelling and weight loss. A majority of the patients had hepatosplenonegaly, ascites and jaundice, and only 6% had metastatic tumors. The duration of the symptoms ranged from 1 month to 16 months with an average of 6 months. In the last decade, it has been established that hepatitis B virus (HBV) infection is the predominant cause of liver disease in the areas of the world where the incidence of PHC is high.[31]

In Atiyeh's study,[30] the evidence suggests a link between the two diseases. Of 54 patients, 30 (55%) were positive for hepatitis B surface antigen (HBsAg), which was higher than in matched controls (18%) or in the general population (8%). Some studies suggest schistosomiasis, a common disease in Saudi Arabia, as an important risk factor for liver cancer.[32] Moulds that produce aflotoxins, notably *Aspergillus flavus,* have a synergistic effect with the HBV in the causation of PHC.[33] Food contamination with fungus has not yet been studied in Saudi Arabia.

ORAL AND PHARYNGEAL CANCERS

Oral and pharyngeal cancers are primarily squamous cell carcinomas, usually well differentiated. Globally, they are among the ten most common cancers. Reported incidence rates around the world vary approximately 15-fold,[34] and the etiological factors vary both geographically and culturally. Data collected from six countries in South East Asia showed a strong association between tobacco chewing and oral cancer.[35] Lesser associations were evident for smoking, alcohol consumption, vitamin A deficiency[36] and Epstein-Barr virus.[37]

In Saudi Arabia the frequency of the cancers varied in the different studies according to location and time. In both Taylor's[2] and Perrine's[4] studies in Aramco Hospital in Dhahran, nasopharyngeal cancer ranks low among other tumors. On the other hand, in the study of El-Akkad[14] in King Faisal Specialist Hospital, Riyadh, it ranked fifth (third among males and tenth among females).

Stirling et al.[6] observed that the distribution of cancer of the gastrointestinal tract is almost the reverse of that encountered in the West, in that cancers of the mouth, tongue and esophagus are more common than cancers of the lower intestinal tract. In a follow-up study, the authors found that cancer of the mouth was the third most common malignancy.

Stirling et al.[38] studied the distribution of 147 oral cancers referred to the Central Laboratory in Jeddah. The ratio of males to females was 2.1 to 1. Eight out of nine patients had a history of using *shamma* which is a mixture of powdered tobacco leaf, carbonate of lime and other substances including ash. It is used as a quid and retained in the buccal cavity. The habit is most prevalent in the southern part of Saudi Arabia especially among men. The Ames test on *Salmonella typhimurium* bacteria proved that *shamma* water extract produced significant mutagenicity, at least 2.5 times the control. Sodium bicarbonate, a constituent of *shamma* deteriorates to the carbonate, a corrosive capable of damaging epithelium and evoking a disturbed growth pattern. It is conceivable that carbonate may act as a co-carcinogen with tobacco.

El-Akkad[1] observed that the frequency of oral cavity cancer in females from Asir (12.9%) was three times that in the country as a whole (4.4%) and in the males it was twice as high (8.2% versus 4.1%). The high frequency of oral cavity cancer in Asir equals the rate in Bombay, one of the highest rates in the world, and 8.5 times the rate in the USA. The author also attributes the problem to the chewing of *shamma*. In a study conducted by Amer et al.,[39] 33 of 68 patients with oral cancer referred to the King Faisal Specialist Hospital admitted to using *shamma*. Of these *shamma* users 85% were referred from the Southern Province particularly from the Gizan area (73%).

A Royal Decree was issued in 1983 prohibiting the use of *shamma*. Further studies are needed to explore etiological factors including the role of vitamin A deficiency and Epstein-Barr virus.

THYROID CANCER

Thyroid cancer is considered a relatively benign cancer which grows slowly but sometimes can be a rapidly fatal disease.

In Saudi Arabia it ranks inconsistently among other tumors. In different studies it ranked fourteenth,[6] thirteenth,[14] and eighth.[1] The incidence was always higher in females than in males. The predominant type was papillary adenocarcinoma followed by the follicular type.[40]

Macaron et al.[40] studied 35 Saudi patients with thyroid cancer (15 males and 20 females) who attended King Faisal Specialist Hospital, Riyadh, during 1976-1978. The most common clinical presentation was that of a thyroid mass or a lump in the neck, usually of considerable size (4-6 cm in diameter), forming a painless, hard, and irregular mass, of 6 months to 20 years duration leading to the pressure symptoms. Hoarseness of the voice, dysphagia, or breathlessness had led the patients to seek medical advice rather than the mass itself. Twenty-six patients had clinical evidence of metastasis. Nodular goiter and previous exposure to radiation therapy were excluded as predisposing factors; endemic goiter is very rare even in mountainous areas. It is possible that solar radiation may be a contributing factor. The authors believed that thyroid carcinoma occurred more frequently in Saudi Arabia than elsewhere.

CANCER OF THE BREAST

In Taylor's study[2] (1950-1961), only eight cases of breast cancer were detected in 193 cancerous patients seen over 12 years. This startling low incidence of breast cancer in early published series was attributed to the resistance of female Saudis to physical examination as in later studies, breast cancer was the most common cancer among females.[1, 6, 14]

Jamjoom[41] reported that 22 women seen at the King Abdul Aziz University Hospital in Jeddah had breast cancer. It was the most common malignancy constituting 14% of the total number of cancers seen in the hospital over a 2-year period (1978-1979). Every third breast condition seen and treated was confirmed as pathological cancer. Patients were relatively young and mostly came in an advanced condition (stages II and IV). On average the duration of history was 6 months. This late presentation was attributed to shyness and fear on the part of the patients as well a to a shortage of medical facilities.

It is a traditional belief that early and multiple pregnancies offer some protection for women against breast cancer but recent investigations have not substantiated this theory.[42] The findings from Saudi Arabia also refute the theory.

CANCER OF THE CERVIX

Twenty-five years ago, the reluctance of Saudi women to undergo medical examinations interfered with the diagnosis of cancer of the cervix. Only one of 193 patients with cancer in Taylor's study[2] had cancer of the cervix. In three studies conducted more recently,[1, 4, 14] cancer of the cervix ranked third to fifth among females. Its frequency in El-Akkad's study was 7.2% which is very moderate when compared to the frequency in other countries such as Lebanon 38%, Iran 21% and Tunisia 18.4%.[14] The diversified effects of multiple pregnancies, low rate of female promiscuity and male circumcision on the prevalence of cancer of the cervix in Saudi Arabia need to be investigated.

LUNG CANCER

Bronchiogenic carcinoma has a high incidence in Western industrialized countries.[18] In the USA it causes about 80,000 deaths each year and is increasing in both men and women with time. The rates are still about four times as high in men as in women.[42] There is no doubt that the main cause of lung cancer is cigarette smoking. The risk of dying of lung cancer is between 8 and 15 times higher among cigarette smokers than among non-smokers. Other predisposing causes include asbestosis, radioactive ore mining, chromate production, nickel refining and general atmospheric pollution.

In Saudi Arabia the frequency of lung cancer has also apparently increased with time. In Taylor's study[2] only five cases were reported in 261 cancerous patients over 12 years (1950-1961), whereas in the 1970s and 1980s lung cancer occupied the second and third position in two different studies.[1, 4] The frequency among males was 5.6 times the frequency among females.[4] This increase of frequency could be attributed to smoking habits specially among young men. Smoking among young women recently became a sign of modernization which - unless checked - might lead to a change in the pattern. The pollution which is increasing in the main cities in Saudi Arabia could also be a contributing factor. Smoking of *sheesha* and its relation to bronchiogenic carcinoma is presently under study.[43] Although there is a general awareness among Saudis of the hazards of smoking, people are still relaxed and fatalistic in their attitudes towards it: "If God wants a person to have cancer he will have it... smoking or not smoking". This fatalistic attitude (which has no sound religious grounds) dictates, in general, many Saudis' outlook towards health and disease.

CANCER OF THE BLADDER

The relation of bladder cancer to aromatic amines, tobacco smoking and coffee consumption has been reported.[44, 45, 46] Carcinoma of the bladder in patients with urinary schistosomiasis could be due to several factors including carcinogens in the urine or depressed immunocompetence caused by the Schistosoma antigen.[47] Cancer of the bladder is common among sufferers of schistosomiasis in Egypt, but is much less common in the Arabian peninsula although the schistosomiasis is endemic.[48]

In Saudi Arabia bladder cancer showed a low frequency in most of the studies conducted so far. However, in a series of 7,251 cases of cancer studied by El-Akkad,[1] the Asir Province stood out as having a higher frequency of bladder cancer among males (6%) compared with the rest of the country (3.7%). The author attributed the difference to the endemicity of schistosomiasis in Asir. Hanash et al.[49] reported bilharzial bladder cancer in 30 out of 40 bladder cancer patients seen at King Faisal Specialist Hospital (1978-1981).

SKIN CANCER

The incidence of skin cancer varies from country to country, with the highest recorded rate in Australia (50% of all cancers), and the lowest in Bombay (3% of all cancers). The incidence of the two main types of skin cancer, basal cell carcinoma and squamous cell carcinoma is directly related to prolonged and continuous exposure to meteorologic and geographic conditions producing great quantities of ultraviolet (UV) radiation.[50] Other possible predisposing factors are arsenic, tar and tropical ulcers.

The intensity of carcinogenic UV radiation varies in different geographical locations depending upon latitude, zenith angle, concentration of stratospheric ozone and other conditions in the atmosphere.[51] Therefore, skin cancer incidence rates vary in different parts of the world.

Saudi Arabia has one of the greatest solar energy intensities in the world,[52] yet data on skin cancer are rather inconsistent. Taylor[2] reported

16 cases (ten squamous and six basal cell) in 264 cancer cases (6%). In his opinion "This is lower than would be expected in an arid desert climate with most Saudis being exposed to the blazing desert sun for a lifetime." However, he attributed this low rate to the short life expectancy of Saudis (being 39 years) whereas skin cancer occurs most frequently in older groups (no reliable demographic data were available).

El-Akkad in one study[14] also reported a low rate of skin cancer (3.4%) — which ranked tenth among other cancers and ranked fourteenth in another study.[1] This low rate was attributed to the cultural habits of avoiding exposure to solar UV radiation and wearing a headdress (*ghutrah, shumach* and veil).

The relative incidence of skin cancers was estimated from the study of a total of 1,296 cancer patients at the King Faisal Specialist Hospital during 1982. Only 2.7% of all cancer patients had cancer of the skin.[53]

Woodhouse (1982)[54] observed that Saudi people have a low body content of vitamin D and that Western expatriates living in the Central Region of Saudi Arabia do not experience sunburning. These observations, in addition to the low incidence of skin cancer, might imply that there are factors, both cultural and environmental, playing a significant role in reducing the biological activities of solar UV radiation. Partial immunity of the Arabs to basal cell cancer has been suggested.[11]

On the other hand, two other studies showed a high incidence of skin cancer in Saudi Arabia. Sayigh *et al.*[55] reviewed data on 3,251 malignancy cases studied over 10 years by the Pathology Department, Central Laboratory in Riyadh. Skin cancer was the third most predominant malignancy (15%) after cancers of the lymphoreticular system (25%) and the gastrointestinal tract (20%). The male to female ratio (1.7 to 1), the increased incidency by age, and the predominant site of facial and scalp lesions, all corresponded with tumor characteristics in other parts of the world. The ratio of squamous cell carcinoma to basal cell carcinoma (2.3 to 1) was somehow inverted from the usual pattern.

Stirling[6] reported a high proportion of skin cancer (15.5%) among 1,000 consecutive malignant neoplasms in Saudi residents in the Western Region of Saudi Arabia. Skin cancer was the most predominant cancer in the series and it was mostly of the squamous cell type.

This discrepancy in the prevalence of skin cancer between the various studies could be due to true differences between regions, or false differences resulting from inconsistency in the methods of data analysis or the nomenclatures used.

Saudi Arabia, with its numerous sunny days, would appear to provide an ideal climate for cutaneous melanoma. However melanoma of the skin is uncommon. Only 22 cases were seen at King Faisal Specialist Hospital between 1975 and 1982 (a denominator was not given). Most of the tumors were on the foot or head, advanced at diagnosis, and were rapidly fatal.[56] Only one case of naevoid basal cell carcinoma was diagnosed at King Khalid University Hospital, Riyadh.[57]

OTHER TYPES OF CANCER

Twenty patients with retinoblastoma (14 boys and six girls) were seen at the King Faisal Specialist Hospital and Research Center during 2 years 1976-1978.[58] Since the survival rate is improving, it is believed that the genetic pool will increase and with it the incidence of retinoblastoma.

From the experience at the King Faisal Specialist Hospital, neuroblastoma was the seventh commonest cancer found in a study of 500 children. The tumor accounted for 4.6% of these childhood cancers and was surpassed in numbers by leukemia, non-Hodgkin's lymphoma, brain tumors, Hodgkin's disease, retinoblastoma and Wilm's tumor.[59]

Malignant small round cell tumor of the thoracopulmonary region in childhood is a rare neoplasm. Only one patient (a 12-year-old Yemeni) was diagnosed out of 736 cases of solid tumors in children seen over 9 years (1976-1985) at the King Faisal Specialist Hospital.[60] Leiomyosarcoma of the colon is a very rare tumor. The first case in Saudi Arabia was reported in 1985.[61]

KNOWLEDGE AND ATTITUDES TOWARDS CANCER

The detection of a malignant neoplasm has a negative effect on the patient's psyche if he or she knows it. Bedikian *et al.* (1985)[62] have studied the attitude of a sample of Saudi patients towards cancer. The study revealed that only 16% of the patients were informed by the physician in charge about the nature of the illness prior to referral to the oncologist. Many patients were misinformed about the disease. For example, 11 patients had avoided sexual contact for fear it might spread the disease, and this resulted in divorce for three couples. The study also showed that sleep disturbance, fear, and sadness were common and were reported by about 40% of patients.

The authors went further to evaluate the need for psychosocial counselling for Saudi cancer patients.[63] Their study of 100 patients (66 males and 34 females) showed that 92% had an adverse reaction to the discovery of cancer. Fear and sadness were the most common reactions. Sleep disturbance, anxiety and sexual dysfunction were quite common, whereas anger, shame and guilt were uncommon (contrary to the experience of Western societies) (Table 4). Women tended to suffer emotional or sleep disturbances more often than men.

In another study,[64] 250 Saudis from the general public were asked their opinions relating to cancer presentation, etiology, diagnosis, and treatment. The study revealed several areas where Saudis were uninformed or misinformed.

The Saudi patients, however, have some advantages over their Western counterparts. They have better family ties which provide psychological support and they do not need to worry about the financial burden of treatment since the government pays for all treatment and rehabilitation.

The Islamic view of the well-being of man with the emphasis on faith in God, trust in His mercy, acceptance without complaint or grievance of whatever befalls, non-surrender to despair, and the belief that true happiness is the happiness in the hereafter, alleviates the impact of pain and sorrow on the Muslim.[65]

Table 4. Emotional Reactions to Cancer in 100 Patients.

Reaction	Number of Patients
Fear	69
Sadness	64
Emotional disturbance	53
Sleep disturbance	47
Powerlessness/worthlessness	34
Shock	32
Anger	25
Social dysfunction	24
Sexual dysfunction	20
Shame	11
Intellectual dysfunction	8
Guilt	1
None of the above	8

From Ref. 63.

Nevertheless, Bedikian (1985)[63] argues that patients should be enlighted about their disease, alleviated of their fears and anxieties, and given counselling for their social difficulties. He bases his argument on the fact that one-third of his patients continued to have psychosocial difficulties a year after they became aware of their diagnosis. The author concluded that a significant amount of suffering could be spared cancer patients if they were provided with opportunities to vent their psychosocial problems. Because several of the patients with potentially curable malignant neoplasms come late for treatment or discontinue their treatment prematurely, it becomes important further to investigate the psychological and social factors that intervene between the patients and their therapy.

The care of terminally ill patients is a problem at present in Saudi Arabia. It is difficult to discharge cancer patients from a hospital and in the meantime there are no nursing homes available. The traditional extended family is gradually changing into a nuclear family which makes a terminally ill patient quite a burden.

WHICH WAY FORWARD?

Cancer in Saudi Arabia is an ever increasing problem as people change their lifestyle and longevity increases. From Aramco Hospital in Dhahran in 1975 came the report "Of all diseases malignancy is, in recent years, the second major cause of death in Saudi Arab employees (cardiovascular disease ranks first). Among Saudi Arab dependents malignancy as a cause of death has varied from second to fifth place."[4]

It is postulated that 50% of deaths from cancer, worldwide, could be prevented if existing medical and scientific knowledge were effectively used.[66] A national cancer registry program is essential to define the rates of morbidity and mortality and to draw a distribution map. Further clinico-epidemiological research should be carried out for better understanding of the etiology, treatment and methods of control. Saudi cancer patients usually seek treatment several months after the beginning of the symptoms.[67] From King Faisal Specialist Hospital records, it seems that more than 70% of the cancer patients are admitted in an advanced stage, usually beyond curative therapy.[15, 62] Therefore, health education programs for public and professionals should promote awareness, early diagnosis and prompt treatment. Precautions should be taken against carcinogenic factors in the environment such as smoking, excessive industrial pollution and exposure to excessive ultraviolet radiation.

The incidence of cancer is estimated at around 800 new cases per million per year (approximately 400 in Kuwait, 1,000 in Iraq and 4,000 in the USA).[68]

Taking into consideration population growth, increase of life expectancy at birth, and industrialization, up to 10,000 new cases per year could be expected soon. Well equipped cancer centers should therefore be planned.

REFERENCES

1. **El-Akkad SM, Amer MH, Lin GS, Sabbah RS, Godwin JT.** Pattern of cancer in Saudi Arabs referred to King Faisal Specialist Hospital. *Cancer* 1986(in press).

2. **Taylor JW.** Cancer in Saudi Arabia. *Cancer* 1963; 16: 1530-1536.

3. **Azar HA.** Cancer in Lebanon and the Near East. *Cancer* 1962; 15:66-78.

4. **Perrine RP, Juma'a A.** Changing trends in cancer in Saudi Arabia. *Epidemiology Bulletin*. Dhahran: Aramco Medical Department, January 1975: 1-4.

5. **Gelpi AP.** Malignant lymphoma in Saudi Arabia. *Cancer* 1970; 25:892-895.

6. **Stirling G, Khalil AM, Nada GN, Saad AA, Raheem MA.** Malignant neoplasm in Saudi Arabia. *Cancer* 1979; 44: 1543-1548.

7. **Stirling GA, Khalil AM, Nada GM, Saad AA, Raheem MA.** A study of one thousand consecutive malignant neoplasms in Saudis 1975-1977. *Saudi Med J* 1979; 1: 89-94.

8. **Bin Ahmed OS, Sabbah RS.** Childhood non-Hodgkin's lymphoma in Saudi Arabia: Clinical features of 100 cases. *King Faisal Specialist Hosp Med J* 1982; 2: 217-224.

9. **Frazer JW.** Malignant lymphomas of the gastrointestinal tract. *Surg Gynec Obstet* 1959; 108: 182-190.

10. **El-Gazayerli M, Kharadly M, Khalil H, Galal R, Raid W, El-Gazayerli MM.** Primary tumours of lymph nodes. In: *Lymphoreticular tumours in Africa* (Symposium). Basel/New York: S. Karger, 1964: 36-41.

11. **Froede RC, Mason JK.** Malignant disease of Aden Arabs. *Cancer* 1965; 18: 1175-1179.

12. **Racoveanu NT.** Cancer activities in WHO Eastern Mediterranean Region during 1976. In: *WHO Second Meeting of the Regional Advisory Panel on Cancer*, Tunis, 18 Nov 1976; Annex IV: 1-7. v.

13. **American Cancer Society:** Cancer statistics, 1985. *Ca-A Cancer J Clinicians* 1985; 35: 19-35.

14. **El-Akkad S.** Cancer in Saudi Arabia: a comparative study. *Saudi Med J* 1983; 4: 156-164.

15. **Amer MH.** Pattern of cancer in Saudi Arabia: A personal experience based on the management of 1,000 patients, Part I. *King Faisal Specialist Hosp Med J* 1982; 2: 203-215.

16. **Koriech OM, Al Kuhaymi R.** Cancer in Saudi Arabia: Riyadh Al-Kharj Hospital Programme Experience. *Saudi Med J* 1984; 5: 217-233.

17. **Aur RJA, Sackey K, Sabbah RS,** *et al.* Combination therapy for childhood acute lymphocytic leukemia. *King Faisal Specialist Hosp Med J* 1985; 5: 79-89.

18. **Waterhouse JAH.** International epidemiology of cancer. *J R Coll Physicians Lond* 1985; 19: 10-12.

19. **Tuyns AJ, Pequignot G, Jenson DM.** Role of diet, alcohol and tobacco in esophageal cancer, as illustrated by two contrasting high-incidence areas in the north of Iran and west of France. *Front Gastrointest Res* 1979; 4: 101-110.

20. **Doll R.** Geographical variation in cancer incidence: a clue to causation. *World J Surg* 1978; 2: 595-602.

21. **Coordinating Group for the Research of Esophageal Carcinoma.** The epidemiology of esophageal cancer in north China and preliminary results in the investigation of its etiological factors. *Chin Med J* 1975; 1: 167-183.

22. **Mellow MH, Layne EA, Lipman TO et al.** Plasma zinc and vitamin A in human squamous carcinoma of the esophagus. *Cancer* 1983: 51: 1615-1620.

23. **Miller RW.** Cancer epidemics in the People's Republic of China. *J Natl Cancer Inst* 1978; 60: 1195-1203.

24. **Munoz N, Grassi A. Qiong S, et al.** Pre-cursor lesions of oesophageal cancer in high-risk populations in Iran and China. *Lancet* 1982; 1: 876-879.

25. **Van Rensburg SJ.** Epidemiologic and dietary evidence for a specific nutritional predisposition to esophageal cancer. *J Natl Cancer Inst* 1981; 67: 243-251.

26. **Al-Karawi M, Al Otaibi R, Kilbane AJ, Yassawy I.** High prevalence of oesophageal carcinoma - results of three-year retrospective study of 1,550 upper gastro-intestinal endoscopies. In: *Proceedings of the 7ᵗʰ Saudi Medical Meeting.* Dammam: King Faisal University, 1982: 248-251.

27. **Shobokshi OA.** Endoscopy of the upper gastrointestinal tract analysis of 551 cases. In: *Proceedings of the 7ᵗʰ Saudi Medical Meeting.* Dammam: King Faisal University, 1980: 879-889.

28. **Amer MH.** Epidemiologic aspects of esophageal cancer in Saudi Arabian patients. *The King Faisal Specialist Hosp Med J* 1985; 5: 69-78.

29. **Monib AEM.** A pilot study of gastrointestinal, pancreatic and liver cancer at King Faisal Hospital, Taif. In: Mahgoub E *et al.* eds. *Proceedings of the 5ᵗʰ Saudi Medical Meeting.* Riyadh: University of Riyadh, 1980: 701-706.

30. **Atiyeh M, Ali MA.** Primary hepatocellular carcinoma in Arabia: a clinical pathological study of 54 cases. *Am J Gastrol* 1980; 74: 25-29.

31. **Blumberg BS, Larouze B, London WT, et al.** The relation of infection with the hepatitis B agent to primary hepatic carcinoma. *Am J Pathol* 1975; 81: 669-682.

32. **Inaba Y, Maruchi N, Matsuda M, Yamamoto S, Yoshihara N.** A case-control study on liver cancer with special emphasis on the possible aetiological role of schistosomiasis. *Int J Epidemiol* 1984; 13: 408-412.

33. **Emmons PR, Harrison MJD, Honour AJ, Mitchell JR.** Hepatitis B and hepatocellular carcinoma. *Lancet* 1978; 6: 218.

34. **McMichael AJ.** Oral cancer in the Third World: time for preventive intervention? *Int J Epidemiol* 1984; 13: 403-405.

35. **Hirayama T.** An epidemiological study of oral and pharyngeal cancer in central and south-east Asia. *Bull WHO* 1966; 34: 41-69.

36. **Ibrahim K, Jafarey NA, Zuberi SJ.** Plasma vitamin 'A' and carotene levels in squamous cell carcinoma of the oral cavity and oro-pharynx. *Clin Oncol* 1977; 3: 203-207.

37. **Ernberg N, Kallin B.** Epstein-Barr virus and its association with human malignant diseases. *Cancer Surveys* 1984; 3: 51-89.

38. **Stirling G, Zahran F, Jamjoom A, Eed D.** Cancer of the mouth in the western region of Saudi Arabia: a histopathological and experimental study. *King Abdulaziz Med J* 1981; 1: 10-16.

39. **Amer M, Bull CA, Daouk MN McArthur, P D, Lundmark GJ, El Senoussi M.** Shamma usage and oral cancer in Saudi Arabia. *Ann Saudi Med* 1985; 5: 135-141.

40. **Macaron C, Ali MA, Berghan R.** King Faisal Specialist Hospital experience in thyroid cancer. In: *Proceedings of the 4th Saudi Medical Conference.* Dammam: King Faisal University, 1980: 751-756.

41. **Jamjoom AM.** Two-years experience in King Abdul Aziz University Hospital, Jeddah, of treatment of advanced cancer of the breast. In: Mahgoub E, *et al.* eds. *Proceedings of the 5th Saudi Medical Meeting.* Riyadh; University of Riyadh, 1980: 619-628.

42. Higgins I. Respiratory disease. In: Last JM, ed. *Maxcy-Rosenau public health and preventive medicine,* 11th ed. New York: Appleton-Century-Crofts, 1980: 1239-1255.

43. **Zahran FM, Baig MHA.** Long term effects of sheesha and cigarette smoking on the respiratory system in Saudi Arabia. In: *Proceedings of the 7th Saudi Medical Meeting.* Dammam: King Faisal University, 1982: 160-165.

44. **Snowdon DA, Phillips RL.** Coffee consumption and risk of fatal cancers. *Am J Public Health* 1984; 74: 820-823.

45. **Mettlin C, Graham S.** Dietary risk factors in human bladder cancer. *Am J Epidemiol* 1979; 110: 255-263.

46. **Anonymous.** Bladder cancer and smoking (Leading article). *Br Med J* 1972; 1:763.

47. **Mee AD.** Aetiological aspects of bladder cancer in urinary bilharzia. *Saudi Med J* 1982; 3: 123-127.

48. **Hicks RM, Walters CL, Elsebai I, El-Aaser** *et al.* Demonstration of nitrosamines in human urine: preliminary observations on a possible etiology for bladder cancer in association with chronic urinary tract infections. *Proc R Soc Med* 1977; 70: 413-7.

49. **Hanash KA, Bissada NK, Abla A** *et al.* Predictive value of excretory urography, ultrasonography, computerized tomography, and liver and bone scan in the staging of bilharzial bladder cancer in Saudi Arabia. *Cancer* 1984; 54: 172-176.

50. **Epstein JH.** *Photocarcinogenesis: a review.* Department of Health, Education and Welfare Publication (NIH) 78-1532, International Conference on Ultraviolet Carcinogenesis. Natl Cancer Inst Monogr 1978; 50: 13-25.

51. **Urbach F.** Welcome and introduction: *Evidence and epidemiology of ultraviolet - induced cancers in man.* International Conference on Ultraviolet Carcinogensis. Natl Cancer Inst Monogr 1978; 50: 5.

52. **Sayigh AAM.** Saudi Arabia and its energy resources. Paper presented at COMPLES Meeting. Dhahran, 1975.

53. **Hannan MA, Paul M, Amer MH, Al-Watban FH.** Study of ultraviolet radiation and genotoxic effects of natural sunlight in relation to skin cancer in Saudi Arabia. *Cancer Res* 1984; 44: 2192-2197.

54. **Woodhouse NJY. Norton WL.** Low vitamin D levels in Saudi Arabians. *King Faisal Specialist Hosp J* 1982; 2: 127-131.

55. **Sayigh AAM, Sebai ZA, Abdul Halim.** Preliminary study of the solar radiation effect on skin cancer. In: *Proceedings of Biological Society of Saudi Arabia.* Riyadh: University of Riyadh, 1977; 185-200.

56. **Mughal T, Robinson WA.** Malignant melanoma of the skin. *King Faisal Specialist Hosp Med J* 1982; 2: 167-174.

57. **Cardoso E, Sundararajan M.** The naevoid basal cell carcinoma syndrome. *Saudi Med J* 1985; 6: 272-276.

58. **Sabbah R, Schimmelpfenning W, Berry D.** Retinoplastoma in Saudi Arabia. In: *Proceedings of the 4th Saudi Medical Conference.* Dammam: King Faisal University, 1980: 744-750.

59. **Sabbah RS.** Childhood cancer in Saudi Arabia: current problems and suggested solutions. *King Faisal Specialist Hosp Med J* 1982; 2: 273-276.

60. **Rifai S, Aur RJA, Akhtar M. et al.** Malignant small round cell tumor of the thoraco-pulmonary region in childhood. *King Faisal Specialist Hospital Med J* 1985; 5: 127-130.

61. **Bakhsh TM, Mira SA, Serafi AA.** Leiomyosarcoma of the colon. *Saudi Med J* 1985; 6: 454-458.

62. **Bedikian AY, Saleh V, Ibrahim S.** Saudi patients and companions attitudes toward cancer. *King Faisal Specialist Hospital Med J* 1985; 5: 17-25.

63. **Bedikian AY, Saleh V.** An evaluation of the need for psychosocial counselling for Saudi cancer patients. *King Faisal Specialist Hosp Med J* 1985; 5: 91-98.

64. **Bedikian AY, Thompson SE.** Saudi Community Attitude Towards Cancer. *Ann Saudi Med* 1985; 5: 161-168.

65. **Kharola AE.** Islamic view of the well-being of man. *J IMA* 1982; 14: 27.

66. **Hanlon JJ, Pickett GE.** Public health administration and practice. 8th ed. St Louis: Times Mirror/Mosby, 1984: 3-21.

67. **El Faraidi AH.** Surgical treatment of carcinoma of the oesophagus. *Saudi Med J* 1979; 1: 35-40.

68. **El-Akkad S.** Plans for cancer care in Saudi Arabia (Leading article). *Saudi Med J* 1982; 3: 71-74.

ROAD TRAFFIC INJURIES

INTRODUCTION

Injuries are amongst the leading causes of death, worldwide, and road injuries (motor vehicle-related injuries) are the most prevailing types. It is a common misconception that injuries in general, and road injuries in particular, are problems of the industrialized world, as they are also prevalent in developing countries. Reports from many developing countries such as Thailand,[1] India,[2] Papua New Guinea,[3] Zimbawe[4] and Uganda[5] indicate a secular increase in mortality rates due to road injuries. In some of these countries the problem has increased several-fold in one generation and has become the leading cause of death among adult males.

There is a relatively high incidence of road injuries in the Arab world compared with many other parts of the world. The Arab population constitutes 3.6% of the world population, possesses 1% of the total number of cars and suffers 4.8% of total deaths due to road injuries.[6]

The Arab Gulf states have experienced rapid socioeconomic development in the last 15 years. As a consequence there has been a rapid increase in motorization, although without a corresponding development of highway education or highway safety measures,[7] which has led to an epidemic of road injuries.

In Kuwait, for example, road injury is considered the leading cause of death for the population as a whole. The motor vehicle-related fatality rate is 50% higher than in the USA and almost three times as high as that in Britain.[8] Similar results are reported from the United Arab Emirates[9] and Qatar.[10] In the Arab Gulf region, fatality rates per 1,000 vehicles range from 2.5 to 10 times higher than those in Europe or North America,[11] although one should be aware that statistics from the developing world are not always complete or 100% reliable.

THE PROBLEMS IN SAUDI ARABIA

Road injuries constitute a major health problem in Saudi Arabia. Nevertheless, the epidemiology of the problem has not been adequately studied and the first results were not published until 1980. At present, only a few reports are available - mostly based on studies carried out in hospitals and local communities

A study undertaken in Asir Province to explore the causes and types of road injuries over 3 years (1975-1977) provided valuable information.[12] The number of road injuries more than doubled from 1975 to 1977 (from 608 cases to 1,230 cases). During the same period the number of registered cars increased about four times, whereas the length of paved roads increased by only 73%.

Every second bed in the surgical ward of Abha General Hospital was occupied by a patient injured in a vehicular accident. Of the total 3,694 patients injured in road accidents and admitted to the six hospitals in the region, 49.6% were 20-39 years of age. Head injuries were the most prevailing type (46%) and caused 82% of the fatalities. An analysis of the causes of injuries, showed that 62% were due to collisions between two moving vehicles. Driver error caused 97% of the injuries (speeding 51% and careless and irresponsible driving 46%). Only 1.1% of the drivers were under the influence of alcohol or drugs.

In 1979, 17,743 road traffic accidents were recorded in Saudi Arabia.[13] As a result, 16,832 patients were admitted to hospitals suffering from severe injuries. More than 90% of the victims were male and more than 60% were between 15 and 45 years of age. The fatality/injury ratio was 1 to 6. As a result of road injuries 1,178 patients with disabling deformities requiring physiotherapy, occupational therapy and/or reconstructive surgery were estimated to be added to the population pool in the Kingdom every year.

Another study on the epidemiology of road injuries was conducted in Qasim region (1980).[14] The study covered 1,106 persons killed or injured in 1 year. Most accidents were caused by drivers aged 18-30 years

— the most dangerous age group for drivers all over the world. Drugs and alcohol played an insignificant role. Of the 593 drivers involved in accidents in Breida City, 45% had no driving license. Pedestrian casualties formed only 11% of the total but pedestrian deaths constituted 19% of the fatalities. The fatality/injury ratio was 1 to 4, which is very high compared with 1 to 50 in Britain. However, one has to consider the possible differences in defining the term injury and the degree of reliability of the data before final judgment can be made. There was a very high rate of vehicular overturn, especially on the highways (40%). Small pickup trucks (wanait) were involved in 54% of the accidents.

Head injuries and spinal cord injuries cause the most serious and disabling results. Complications include neurological disorders, *respiratory* complications, loss of bowel and bladder function, ulcers, and death from renal or respiratory failure.

In the period 1978-1982 all cases of head injuries admitted to three hospitals in Jeddah,[15] Taif[16] and Al Khobar[17] were studied. The findings showed that motor vehicle-related accidents were the main cause (ranging from 56% to 78%). The injuries were, in general, moderate to severe. The average time of transportation from the scene of the accident to the hospital was about an hour and medical care provided before arrival in hospital was less than adequate.

In the Taif study, road accidents caused 85% of all deaths due to head injury.[16] In the Jeddah study, 66% of the victims had impaired consciousness or were comatose at the time of admission. In Jeddah and Taif, similar to the findings in the Qasim study, the pickup truck (wanait) was responsible for the majority of deaths.

In 1979, an 18-bed Spinal Cord Injury Unit was established in Riyadh Central Hospital.[18] During the first year 72 patients with traumatic spinal cord injuries were admitted. The majority of victims were young adults involved in road traffic accidents often occurring during the seasons of long trips to Makkah at Hajj or Omra time. The average hospital stay was 93 days (ranging from 3 to 330 days). Of the 26 tetraplegic patients, 11 (43%) died. The author concluded that non-use of safety seat belts contributed to the number of spinal injuries.

THE PRESENT SITUATION (1980S)

From the records of the General Traffic Department in Saudi Arabia[19] the following data are indicative:

1. The number of registered cars in Saudi Arabia increased from 144,768 in 1971 to 2,514,115 in 1984 (an annual increase of 126%). The distribution of cars in the regions is shown in Table 1.

2. In 1984, there were 27,384 accidents, 21,850 injured persons and 3,038 deaths in Saudi Arabia. This indicates a very great problem when compared with the statistics of the 1970s.[13] Table 2 shows the distribution of accidents, injuries and deaths according to region.

3. Sixty-four per cent of the accidents occurred during the daytime, 73% were in the main cities, and 85% were caused by human error. Fifty-eight per cent of the cars were sedans, 24% were pickup trucks (wanaits), and 18% were other types. Of the 45,984 drivers, 29% were between 18 and 30 years of age, 53% were Saudis and 37% did not carry licenses.

Several studies on road injuries have been conducted at Riyadh Central Hospital which has a trauma center. The results are indicative of the magnitude and seriousness of the problem. Fatalities due to road accidents mostly occurred either at the scene of the accident or during transportation to the hospital.[20] Over a 4-year period (1980-1983) 92,411 persons were hospitalized, 12,451 (14%) of whom were victims of vehicular accidents — the major cause of fatalities in the hospital (20.7%) followed by cardiovascular disease (13.5%), cerebrovascular disease (12.6%) and malignant neoplasms (10.6%).[20]

Table 1. Number of Cars Registered in Saudi Arabia at the End of 1984 According to Region.

Region	No.	Percentage
*Makkah	864,052	34
Riyadh	676,908	27
Eastern	431,550	17
Qasim	117,593	5
Asir	101,765	4
Madinah	83,102	3
Others	239,145	10
Total:	**2,514,115**	**100**

*Makkah Region covers Jeddah, Makkah and Taif districts.
From Ref. 19.

Over an 18-month period (1983-1984), 565 cases with severe injuries due to road traffic accidents were admitted to the Intensive Care Multiple Trauma units.[21] Almost 60% had multiple injuries sustaining 895 injuries to different parts of the body. The causes of severe injuries were the non-use of safety measures in the car and inadequate management at the scene of the accident or during transportation to the hospital.

Chest injuries can be dramatic and, if not properly and promptly managed, may result in a series of complications. In Riyadh Central Hospital between 1,500 and 2,000 patients with chest injuries are admitted every year. Experience during 7 years showed a sharp increase in the number and severity of chest trauma patients, over 90% of which were due to road traffic accidents.[22]

Table 2. Number and Percentage of Accidents, Injuries and Deaths in 1984 According to Region.

Region	Accidents		Persons Injured		Deaths	
	No.	%	No.	%	No.	%
Riyadh	11,932	43.6	4,553	20.8	389	12.8
Makkah	5,953	21.8	7,514	34.4	1,047	34.5
Asir	1,887	6.9	392	1.8	58	1.9
Eastern	1,419	5.2	1,987	9.1	395	13.0
Qasim	1,194	4.4	1,515	6.9	234	7.7
Tabuk	1,127	4.1	496	2.3	80	2.6
Madinah	1,048	3.8	1,497	6.9	288	9.5
Gizan	1,004	3.7	1,327	6.5	177	5.8
Others	1,785	6.5	2,469	11.3	370	12.2
Total:	**27,348**	**100**	**21,850**	**100**	**3,038**	**100**

From Ref. 19.

In 1980, the rate of traffic deaths in Saudi Arabia was 228 per 100,000 cars[23] which is too high when compared to other industrialized countries such as the USA (42), UK (44), Japan (49), and France (71).[24] Another study, however, suggested that accidents in Saudi Arabia are not more serious than in other countries in terms of injuries and fatalities, as accidents involving only minor injuries or none at all are rarely reported. Since insurance coverage is not compulsory, involved parties tend to settle their financial losses without reporting to the traffic police department, which may explain the very high fatality injury ratio in Saudi Arabia compared with other countries.

THE SOCIOECONOMIC IMPACT OF ROAD INJURIES

Road injuries, fatal or non-fatal, can cause a great strain on the economic resources of the victim, his family and the nation as a whole. Patients often develop a variety of disorders including motor, sensory, vascular, sexual and psychological dysfunctions.

It is not easy to estimate accurately the cost of road injuries to the nation. However, the figure is formidable if the direct and indirect costs are considered. These involve mobilization of patients, lengthy hospitalization time (the average hospital stay can be well over 40 days[25]) and rehabilitation programs. Loss of productivity due to absence from work and physical impairment adds to the problem.

Premature loss of life is a drain on human resources especially in a situation where the victims are mostly adult males in their prime time of life for economic productivity. Consideration must also be given to the cost of damaged property (cars and other objects) and administration of road traffic control.

A trial was made in 1979 to calculate the ultimate cost of 17,743 road traffic accidents in Saudi Arabia which resulted in the hospital admission of 16,832 injured patients (including 1,178 disabled patients requiring further physiotherapy and/or reconstructive surgery) and 2,871 deaths. It was estimated that the country had lost SR 4,776,836 per day (over 16 billion SR per year).[13] By 1986 the figure must be much higher if one considers the increase in population, rate of injuries and cost of treatment.

DISCUSSION

Road injuries in Saudi Arabia as well as in other Arab Gulf states are a major problem. According to Al-Rodhan and Lifeso,[26] "there is an epidemic of road traffic accidents in Saudi Arabia that is second only to infectious diseases as a medical problem. It is an epidemic as serious as plague or smallpox were to earlier generations".

The rate of traffic deaths per 100,000 is high even when compared with industrialized countries.

The rapid socioeconomic development has made the purchase of a car possible for most of the population. It has become accepted for a teenager from a middle class family to obtain a personal car before completing high school. Many of the drivers, as the studies show, are unlicensed. Almost any middle income expatriate can afford to buy a car within a few months of his stay in the country. A used car costs less than SR 7000, an equivalent to 2 month's salary for a clerk.

A Bedouin, newly migrant to the city, would make buying a car his top priority. A joke — which reflects a reality — tells of a young Bedouin who went to buy a car and asked the salesman to direct it in the direction of the main road before he sat — for the first time in his life — behind the steering wheel. The transport for a Bedouin in the desert is usually a pickup truck to move the animals, water and folded tents. Bedouin women drive cars in the desert, in contrast to city women who do not enjoy this privilege.

The rate of fatality is high. The very large number of cars has surpassed facilitative measures such as road engineering or traffic law enforcement. Over 90% of the accidents are due to driver error including speeding, careless driving, ignoring road signs or traffic lights, and driving on the wrong side of the road. Speed is the major cause of accidents in Saudi Arabia. It was the cause of 54%, 64%, 67% and 67% respectively, of the total number of accidents for the successive years 1977 to 1980.[27]

In the early 1980s there were no indications that drugs played a significant role in accidents but there is now a general feeling that they do. Until a few years ago, safety belts were not required to be fitted in cars imported to Saudi Arabia. Now they are, but the population is not aware of their value in preventing or mitigating the seriousness of injuries. Equally important is the lack of public awareness of the value of defensive driving.

In conclusion, road injuries besides being a major health hazard leading to a high rate of morbidity, disability and death, have a great socioeconomic impact on the victim, his family and the nation as a whole. The problem is tractable, and the toll could be greatly reduced if appropriate measures were taken.

WHICH WAY FORWARD?

"The vast numbers of those maimed and killed on the roads are too often accepted fatalistically as a normal part of modern life. Yet, if traffic accidents are tackled by methods like those used against the great killing diseases, the present epidemic of road deaths can be made to diminish just as epidemics of plague and smallpox have now been almost completely eliminated everywhere in the world."[28]

As for many other public health problems the solution to road injuries does not lie in one magic procedure but rather in a series of concomitant actions, the most important of which are listed below.

1. An intelligent use of mass media and educational programs is required to make the public aware of correct driving behavior, defensive driving, and the use of safety belts. Licencing is for the safety of the people rather than to satisfy the interest of the police department.

2. Technical measures have proved to be of more value in accident prevention than attempts to change human behavior.[29] These should be enforced if necessary. Prophet Mohammad — peace be upon Him — said, "God enforces matters by the power of law when the Koran teaching does not effect". The law enforcement of safety belts deserves serious consideration. Such laws have already been passed in many industrialized countries, and safety belts have reduced the severity of injuries in car accidents by 50%.[30] Safety belts and other safety features are estimated to have prevented more than 25,000 deaths in the USA between 1966 and 1975.[31] Air bags also proved to be effective in reducing the severity of injuries.[32]

3. Implementation of child-restraining systems could decrease disability injuries by 78%.[33]

4. Speed limits should be enforced by law. In Britain during the period of November 1973 to July 1975 (the oil crisis period) the speed limit was reduced from 70 to 50 miles per hour in order to save energy. The result was a significant reduction of the injury rate on motorways which reverted to its previous level when the speed limit was raised after the oil crisis.[34]

5. Experience from Denmark has shown that lowered speed limits on the roads are more effective than any other safety measure in reducing the number of deaths and injuries caused by traffic accidents.[35] In November 1973 a speed limit of 80 km per hour on roads outside urban areas was introduced to save petrol during the oil crisis. The number of people killed in road

accidents fell from 1,132 in 1973 to 766 in 1974, a reduction of nearly 33%.

6. Considerable information is available on the undesirable consequences of teenage driving, the over-involvement of teenagers in crashes, their high death rates both as drivers and passengers, and injuries sustained by others involved in crashes with teenage drivers.[36] In the USA motor vehicle crashes are the major cause of death among teenagers,[37] and considerable illegal or deviant teenage driving has been found including unlicensed driving, speeding and driving after drinking. Ways to reduce the high crash rate involving teenage drivers need to be pursued.

7. Although driving licenses are issued at the age of 18, about 40% of the drivers are unlicenced.[14, 19, 27] It should be clearly laid down that driving without a valid license constitutes a serious offence. Furthermore, traffic laws are unfortunately not very clear and regulations regarding enforcement are rather loose. Stricter measures regarding the enforcement of these laws have to be applied. Driving schools must be expanded and improved.

8. A most powerful measure would be compulsory comprehensive vehicle insurance which should suit our culture and Islamic values. This would cost the state nothing. Fiscal penalties for misbehavior would be imposed by the insurance companies. The possession of both valid insurance cover and a valid license is necessary in most developed countries.

9. Deaths from injuries occur to a large extent at the site of the accident or during transportation to the hospital. The need to train drivers and ambulance attendants in proper emergency medical care and life-saving procedures cannot be overemphasized. Rehabilitation and trauma centers are needed in major cities to prepare the disabled for a productive life.[38]

10. More research is needed to study the etiology and epidemiology of road traffic accidents and measures to control the problem. The King Abdul Aziz Research City (previously known as SANCST) is sponsoring research work on the subject; this initiative needs to be supported by other institutions.

REFERENCES

1. **Punyahotra V.** Epidemiology of road traffic accidents in Thailand (1980). National Accident Research Center, National Safety Council of Thailand, 1982.

2. Anonymous. *Major issues in road traffic safety*. Conference on Road Traffic Accidents in Developing Countries, Mexico City, 9-13 November, 1981. Geneva: World Health Organization.

3. **Wyatt BG.** The epidemiology of road accidents in Papua New Guinea. *Papua New Guinea Med J* 1980; 23: 60-65.

4. **Humphries SV.** Seven million casualties. *Central Afr J Med* 1977; 23: 86-88.

5. **Drury RAB.** The mortality of elderly Ugandan Africans. *Trop Geog Med* 1972; 24: 385-392.

6. **Baker SP, Sebai ZA, Haddon W.** Injuries due to accidents: an epidemiological study. *J Jordanian Med* 1976; 11: 15-22 (Arabic).

7. **Wintemute G.** *The size of the problem. In: principles for injury prevention in developing countries.* Geneva: World Health Organization, 1985.

8. *Bayoumi A.* The epidemiology of fatal motor vehicle accidents in Kuwait. *Accidents Analysis and Prevention* 1981; 13: 339-48.

9. **Weddell JM, McDougall A.** Road traffic injuries in Sharjah. *Int J Epidemiol* 1981; 10: 155-159.

10. **Eid AM.** Road traffic accidents in Qatar: the size of the problem. *Accidents Analysis and Prevention* 1980; 12: 287-298.

11. **Ashi JM, El-Desouky M.** *Traffic accidents in the Arab Gulf States.* Secretariat General of Health for the Arab Countries of the Gulf Area, 1981: 99 pp.

12. **Tamimi TM, Daly M, Bhatty MA, Lutfi AHM.** Causes and types of road injuries in the Asir Province, Saudi Arabia, 1975-1977: preliminary study. *Saudi Med J* 1980; 1: 249-256.

13. Anonymous, Socioeconomic impact of road traffic accidents in Saudi Arabia (editorial). *Saudi Med J* 1980; 1: 246-8.

14. **Hamour BA.** Epidemiology of road accidents. In: Sebai ZA, ed. *Community Health in Saudi Arabia*, Jeddah: Tihama Publications, 1984: 45-50.

15. **Tawfik OM, Bakhotma MA, Sulaiman SI.** Head injuries in Jeddah — an analytical study of 200 cases. *Saudi Med J* 1985; 6: 25-34.

16. **Khan AA, Mohiuddin MG.** Head injury in Taif — a review of 1,285 cases — a three-year evaluation. In: *Proceedings of the 7th Medical Meeting.* Dammam: King Faisal University, 1982: 669-673.

17. **El-Meshad MH.** Two years' experience in the management of head injuries in Al-Khobar city. In: *Proceedings of the 7th Medical Meeting.* Dammam: King Faisal University, 1982: 674-77.

18. **Khawashki MI, Abdel-Hafez Y, Chabara AR.** Spinal cord injuries. In: Mahgoub ES, ed. *Proceedings of the 5th Medical Meeting.* Riyadh: University of Riyadh, 1981; 589-608.

19. **Al-Saif A.** *System and organization development of traffic administration: theoretical and experimental aspects.* Riyadh: Isha'a Press 1986: 31-39 (Arabic).

20. **Al-Mofarreh MA, Al-Bunyan AM, Ashoor MT, Markakis EJ.** Fatalities in Riyadh Central Hospital with special reference to road traffic accidents. In: *Proceedings of the 8th Saudi Medical Meeting,* Riyadh, 1983: National Guard Medical Department (in press).

21. **Markakis EJ, Youssef A.** RTA injuries as seen in the multiple trauma unit and ICU in Riyadh Central Hospital. In: *Proceedings of the 8th Saudi Medical Meeting,* Riyadh 1983; National Guard Medical Department (in press).

22. **Hamdy MG.** Chest injuries at Riyadh Central Hospital. In: *Proceedings of the 7th Saudi Medical Meeting.* Dammam: King Faisal University, 1982: 710-15.

23. *Ten years traffic accidents 1971-1980.* An official report. Kingdom of Saudi Arabia: General Traffic Department, Public Security. Ministry of Interior.

24. *Carnage on the highways: how U.S. record compares.* US News and World Report, 1981; 78.

25. **Asogwa SE.** Road traffic accidents: the doctor's point of view. *Afr J Med Medical Sci* 1978; 7: 29-35.

26. **Al-Rodhan N, Lifeso RM.** Traffic accidents in Saudi Arabia: an epidemic. (Special communication). *Ann Saudi Med* 1986; 6: 69-70.

27. **Mufti MH.** Road traffic accidents as a public health problem in Riyadh, Saudi Arabia. *J Traffic Med* 1983; 11: 65-9.

28. **Kaprio LA.** Death on the road. *World Health,* October 1975; 4-9.

29. **Levi L.** Autosclerosis. *World Health* 1975: 10-14.

30. **Sabey BE, Grant BE, Hobbs CA.** *Alleviation of injuries by use of seat belts.* Transport and Road Research laboratory Report 1977: SR 289.

31. **Robertson LS.** *Accidents analysis and prevention* 1977; 9: 151.

32. Anonymous. *The highway loss reduction status report.* Washington DC: Insurance Institute for Highway Safety, 1975; 20: 1-8.

33. **Meyer RJ.** Save the child: children and automobile restraints (Editorial). *Am J Pub Hlth* 1981; 71: 122-123.

34. **Scott PP, Barton AJ.** The effects on road accident rates of the fuel shortage of November, 1973 and consequent legislation. Transport and Road Research Laboratory Supplementary Report (United Kingdom) 1976: 239.

35. **Egsmose L. Egsmose T.** Speed limits save lives. *World Health Forum* 1985; 6: 246-247.

36. **Karpf RS, Williams AF.** Teenage drivers and motor vehicle deaths. *Accidents Analysis and Prevention* 1983; 15: 55-63.

37. **Williams AF, Lund AK, Preusser DF.** Driving behavior of licensed and unlicensed teenagers. *J Pub Hlth Policy* 1985; 6: 379-393.

38. **Malaika S.** The value of a trauma center. In: *8th Saudi Medical Conference* Abstracts. Riyadh, Saudi Arabia: Saudi Arabian National Guard, 1983; 89-90.

CHAPTER II

HEALTH SERVICES

The most important theme in the health services system in Saudi Arabia today is the development of primary health care and health manpower.

This theme is discussed in three sections: an overview; primary health care; and health manpower.

AN OVERVIEW

THE ACHIEVEMENTS OF THE PAST

In 1949 there were 111 physicians and about 1,000 hospital beds in the whole Kingdom of Saudi Arabia. The country, however, has witnessed lately a spectacular development in health services and health manpower.

During the last 15 years (1970-1985) the number of hospitals increased 2.4 times, hospital beds 3.4 and health centers 3 times (Tables 1, 2).[1] During the same period the number of physicians increased from 1,172 to 14,335 (12 times) and the number of nurses from 3,261 to 29,896 (9 times). Figure 1 shows the increase in the Ministry of Health Budget from SR 183 million in 1970 to SR 9,057 million in 1985. The Ministry of Health budget as a percentage of government budget has increased from 2.3% in 1980 to 4.4% in 1985.

The history of organized preventive health services began in the early 1950s with the malaria control program initiated jointly by the Ministry of Health, ARAMCO (Arabian-American Oil Company) and the World Health Organization. This was followed by a series of control programs for schistosomiasis, leishmaniasis, trachoma, tuberculosis and diarrheal diseases. In the 1980s the primary health care concept, adopted by the Alma Ata meeting in 1978, was recognized by the Ministry of Health and became part of its policy.

Health services became available almost everywhere in the country and within the reach of almost every individual. The quality of the services has also improved especially at the tertiary level. Several hospitals of highly advanced technology were established and interventions such as open heart surgery, kidney transplantation, and advanced cancer therapy successfully carried out. Travelling abroad for tertiary medical care, which was the pattern in the past, became almost unnecessary.

Several achievements have also been attained in the field of medical education (pp. 159-165). Medical research has also been initiated. The number of papers published in the last 10 years exceeded the total number published previously. The *Saudi Medical Journal* (established in 1979), and other journals issued by health services agencies and educational institutes have helped in promoting research activities. King Abdul Aziz City for Science and Technology alone has supported 41 medical research projects since its establishment in 1977.

THE CHALLENGE OF THE PRESENT

The country is divided into 11 health regions (Fig. 2); each is headed by a regional health director. The Ministry of Health provides almost 60% of the health services (67% of the hospital beds, 59% of physicians and 54% of the nurses). About 25% of the services are provided by more than 10 different

Figure 1. The development of the budget of the Ministry of Health over 15 years (1970-1985)

The Budget x SR Million

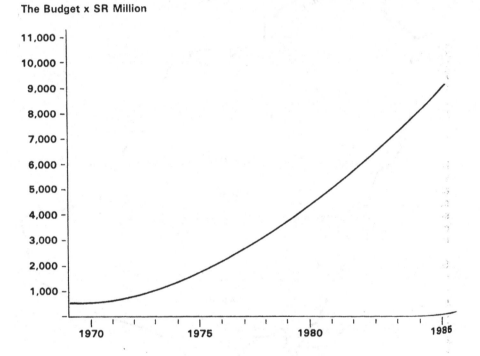

Figure 2. Health Regions in Saudi Arabia

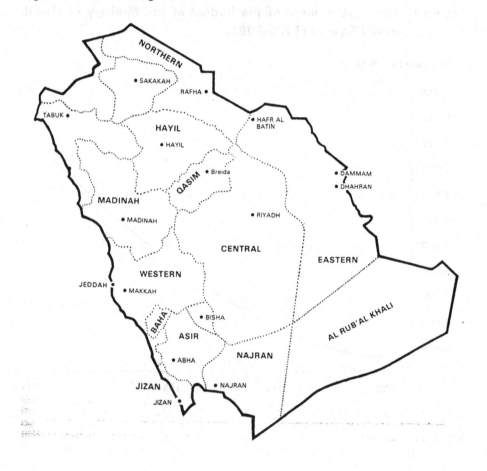

Table 1. Development of Hospitals, Hospital Beds and Health Centers over 15 Years (1970-1985) (governmental and private sectors).

Year	Hospitals	Hospital Beds	Health Centers
1970	74	9,039	591
1971	75	9,837	599
1972	80	10,101	621
1973	85	10,919	667
1974	90	11,161	730
1975	98	12,111	792
1976	99	12,232	903
1977	100	13,346	972
1978	105	13,745	1,042
1979	107	15,582	1,088
1980	109	17,547	1,185
1981	116	18,849	1,263
1982	119	20,775	1,412
1983	126	22,444	1,558
1984	138	23,393	1,633
1985	177	30,707	1,821

From Ref. 1.

Table 2. Development in the Number of Hospitals, Hospital Beds and Health Centers (1970-1985).

	1970	1985
Hospitals		
Ministry of Health	47	104
Other agencies	27	73
Total	**74**	**177**
Hospital beds		
Ministry of Health	7,165	20,463
Other agencies	1,874	10,244
Total	**9,039**	**30,707**
Health centers		
Ministry of Health	519	1,299
Other agencies	72	522
Total	**591**	**1,821**

Modified from Ref. 1

governmental agencies including: The Ministries of Education, Higher Education, Defence and Aviation, the Interior, the National Guard, Girls Education, King Faisal Specialist, King Khalid Eye Hospital, Royal Commission for Jubail and Yanbu, the Red Crescent Society and Aramco (Arabian-American Oil Company) and 15% of the services are provided by the private sector. The governmental health services are free of charge and available to Saudis and non-Saudis also with very few restrictions.

The Ministry of Health budget for the fiscal year 1985-1986 was 9.06 billion (4.4% of the total governmental budget). The governmental expenditure on health (including the Ministry of Health and other governmental agencies) is estimated at SR 15.4 billion, i.e. SR 1,570 per capita expenditure on health by the governmental sector alone (about US$ 420 per capital per year). This is a very high expenditure rate compared to less than US$ 10 per capita per year spent by many developing countries (Table 4). In Zaire for example, primary health care is provided for less than US$ 1 per capita per year.[2]

The rapid growth in the health services system and the diversity of its sources brought quality and a wide coverage of health care also brought some problems, mainly:

1.   The physical development has outgrown the ability for proper planning and management, and the capacity to produce sufficient numbers of Saudi health professionals.
2.   The system has become predominantly curative.
3.   The health information system lags behind.

PLANNING AND MANAGEMENT

More than 10 governmental agencies share responsibility for the provision of health care with the Ministry of Health. They constitute a pool of resources which demands solid planning and coordination. A study sponsored by the Ministry of Planning[3] found that there is an inadequate collaboration between health providers. Only to a certain extent does the Ministry of Health receive information from other health suppliers.

A study of the health services in Asir region[4] showed a centralized system where each of the 115 units (hospitals, health centers, dispensaries and health stations) reported directly to the office of the regional director (Fig. 3). Recently, however, measures have been taken to decentralize the services. As is the case in many other developing countries, the health resources are unevenly distributed between urban and rural areas.

The high expenditure on health services does not seem to have had a maximum impact on health indices. Table 3 compares Saudi Arabia with some selected countries in terms of gross national product (GNP) per capita and infant mortality rate (IMR) per 1,000 live births.[5] In a recent UNICEF study,[6] Saudi Arabia was given as an example of a country with a high infant mortality rate (110 per 1,000 live births) and a high GNP per capita (US$ 12,600). According to the study the high IMR puts Saudi Arabia in the position of a country with GNP per capita of US$ 460.

Figure 3. Organization of the health services in the South Western Region of Saudi Arabia (1980).

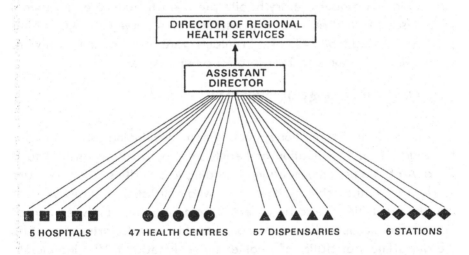

These examples indicate the need to improve the utilization of health resources.

Table 3. Comparison Between Saudi Arabia and Some Selected Countries in Gross National Product Per Capita and Infant Mortality Rate (IMR) Per 1,000 Live Births (1983).

	GNP Per Capita US$	IMR
Saudi Arabia	12,230	65
Sri Lanka	330	39
Malaysia	1,860	30

| Costa Rica | 1,020 | 19 |
| Singapore | 6,620 | 9 |

From Ref. 5.

CURATIVE VS PREVENTIVE SERVICES

With the economic boom in Saudi Arabia many hospitals were expanded, physically improved or newly established. The state of unbalance between curative and preventive services which existed in the past has continued. According to an official report in 1984[3] 'The health services available to the general population are predominantly oriented towards curative services. This curative tendency is even apparent in the primary health sector where mother and child care, antenatal care, information on proper dietary habits, prophylactic routine examinations of pre-school children, etc. are insufficient. A survey of 4,024 out-patients[3] showed that 94% of all contacts were for treatment, 4% were for preventive action and 2% were for other actions.

THE HEALTH INFORMATION SYSTEM

The inefficient information systems in many developing countries makes the planning and evaluation of health services a rather difficult task. Saudi Arabia is not an exception. According to a WHO study[7] 'There are no clear indications on why, how, or by whom statistics of health services and their activities are to be collected, compiled, and analyzed... much information is collected more than once on different departments and by the department of statistics.' Another study[3] noted that 'The incomplete information is a problem in all health agencies'.

Table 4. The Diagnoses of 1,787 Patients made by Three Physicians during 1 Week in Turaba Health Center (1980)

Diagnosis	No.	%
Gastrointestinal diseases	242	13.5
Chest diseases	271	15.2
Cardiovascular diseases	28	1.6
Nervous system diseases	45	2.5
Eye diseases	111	6.2

ENT diseases	160	9.0
Bone and muscle disease	356	19.9
Skin diseases	151	8.4
Genitourinary diseases	87	4.9
Infectious diseases	22	1.2
Common cold	154	8.6
Others	160	9.0
Total	**1,787**	**100.0**

From Ref. 8.

Diagnoses of out-patients attending hospitals and health centers are usually recorded according to the affected organ or the main complaint. Table 4 shows an example from Turaba health center.[8] Apparently such a recording system does not help in understanding the problem, planning for an action or monitoring activities.

The discrepancies in infant mortality rate, as reported by different sources, is an example of the lack of accuracy in vital statistics. Infant mortality rate per 1,000 live births was reported for the period 1982-1984 as 65 by UNICEF,[5] 86 by WHO,[9] 100 by UNICEF,[10] 110 by UNICEF,[6] and 152 in a Milbank Memorial Fund Study.[11] The only available figures of IMR, based on field surveys, were 134 reported in 1969[12] and 117 to 144 reported in 1981.[13] The two field surveys, however, were carried out retrospectively in rural communities and do not represent the country as a whole.

PROMISES FOR THE FUTURE

The future development of health services in Saudi Arabia is a political commitment. The goals of the Fourth Development Plan (1985-1990)[14] were defined as:

1. to improve the quality of health services;
2. to promote comprehensive health care;
3. to strengthen primary health care;
4. to enhance community self reliance; and
5. to further develop health manpower.

The objectives of the plan were stated as follows:

1. to strengthen primary health care as the basis of a comprehensive health services network providing integrated health services of high quality for the people of the Kingdom;
2. to increase the coordination between the Ministry of Health and other agencies that provide health services, and expand exchanges of expertise between the Kingdom and international health organizations;
3. to develop further the health services manpower of the Kingdom at all levels;
4. to continue the development of preventive, public health, and environmental health programs, including health education, maternal and child health care, improved public communication, and occupational health programs;
5. to develop further emergency medical services with special attention to the requirements of the Hajj season; and
6. to continue encouraging the expansion of private health care programs and promote private sector participation in all health services.

The Fourth Development Plan (1985-1990) has wisely shifted the emphasis towards more balanced health services. 'During the Fourth Plan emphasis will be placed increasingly on the balanced growth of primary health services, according to both regional needs and those of specific groups within society. The benefits of maternal and child health care and improved diagnostic services will be made accessible to both urban and rural areas, while emergency services to assist victims of road traffic accidents will also be strengthened.'[14] The Fourth Plan made a special reference to the importance of information systems and research for health development. 'As services and facilities expanded in the Third Plan period, it became essential to ensure that these services operate with maximum efficiency and effectiveness. To accomplish this task, an effective health information system must be established for the continuous evaluation of health services, including those provided by the private sector... in order to achieve a balanced and integrated health services network.'[14]

Health manpower development received a special consideration in the Fourth Plan 'The growth of secondary services in the Third Plan period, and the expansion of primary health centers anticipated in the Fourth Plan period, make it essential that the effectiveness of doctors working for primary health centers, and of technical personnel in the health network, be up-graded.'[14]

With an appreciation of the achievements in the past, and a consideration of the political commitment and the potential resources available, the future of the Kingdom's health services looks promising.

PRIMARY HEALTH CARE

The present situation and the future perspective of primary health care (PHC) in Saudi Arabia cannot be separated from the global situation.

AN INTERNATIONAL PERSPECTIVE

International Conference on Primary Health Care, held in 1978 at Alma Ata, expressed the need for urgent action by all governments, health and development workers, and the world community to protect the health of all the people of the world.[15] The declaration of the meeting stated that 'A main social target of governments, international organizations, and the whole world community should be attainment by all the people of the world by the year 2000, of a level of health that will permit them to lead socially and economically productive lives. Primary health care is the key to this target.'

The declaration went on to define primary health care (PHC) as:

1. essential health care based on practical, scientifically sound, and socially acceptable methods;
2. care that addresses the main health problems in the community by providing promotive, preventive, curative and rehabilitative services; and

3.   care that encompasses health education, the promotion of increased food supplies, proper nutrition, an adequate supply of safe water, basic sanitation, maternal and child health care, and the prevention and control of common diseases and injuries.

Eight years have already passed since the Alma Ata meeting, and with 14 years remaining in this century, one has to ponder whether the goal of health for all in the year 2000 through primary health care is achievable especially in the developing world.

The warning message given by the General Director of the World Health Organization on the health situation of the world in 1981 is quite alarming.[16] The message states the following:

1.   Four-fifths of the world's population have no permanent form of health care.
2.   The threat posed by such major diseases as malaria, schistosomiasis, filariasis, trypanosomiasis, leishmaniasis, cholera, and leprosy either has not lessened in recent years or has actually increased. Almost a quarter of the world's population remains infected with worms.
3.   Only one in three persons in developing countries has reasonable access to safe water and adequate sanitation.
4.   Infant mortality rates remain high in all developing countries and the rate of improvement has begun to slacken.
5.   More than five million children annually defecate themselves to death.
6.   More than half of all child deaths can be traced to the vicious complex of malnutrition and diarrheal and respiratory diseases.
7.   A newborn child in some African countries has only a 50% chance of survival to adolescence.

The Director of 'Health for All' (WHO) estimated that fewer people have access to primary health care now than 5 years ago, except in certain countries and certain parts of countries.[17] The reasons for this unhealthy situation include financial problems, ineffective management, the irrational use of resources, and the inappropriate training of health personnel.

It is well known that primary health care, if delivered properly, can meet almost 80% of the health needs of the people and only 20% of health problems should be referred to secondary and tertiary health care. However, throughout the world primary health care is predominantly curative in nature, with minimum preventive or promotive aspects. Some countries have started pioneering primary health care projects with a comprehensive health care approach. Among them are the West Azerbaijan Project in Iran,[18] Etimesgut Health District in Turkey,[19] rural health project in Guatemala,[20] the Karaiba Experimental Project in Sudan (Sebai, personal observation) and the Loiza Primary Health Care Center in Puerto Rico (Sebai, personal observation). Most of these projects, years after their establishment, still remain experimental. They were started as vertical programs, lacking the means to expand and become integrated with the health system.

What about the future? Statistics tell us that most of the world's population does not have access to basic health services. In many developing countries less than US$10 per person per year is being spent on health (the 25 poorest countries in the world spent an average of US$1.70 in 1980) (Table 14). The number of malnourished children is expected to increase by 30% by the turn of the century. The approach to health sector development in general is fragmented and irrational. A WHO survey carried out in 70 of 134 countries that signed the Alma Ata decree showed that most of them find it difficult to live up to their commitment.[21] In a progress report on the global situation in 1984[22] it was found that a high level of political sensitization has taken place but few countries have well-defined plans of action that include specific objectives, a time frame, and data on the projection and allocation of resources.

One wonders what magic could change the situation in a period of 14 years to achieve the goal of health for all by the year 2000. Is the economy of the developing world going to improve and is more money going to be available to the health sector? Is the political commitment of the 134 member states of the WHO that signed the Alma Ata decree going to be fulfilled, so that health will be considered an objective of economic development? Are health authorities and medical educators going to change their approach to health care from focusing on individual patient care to a holistic approach to health? How can the dream be turned into a reality?

What is needed is not technical knowledge, but political commitment, wise utilization of resources, proper training of health manpower, awakening people's awareness of their actual health needs and efficient management. For the dream to be turned into a reality, all political, economical and educational decisions should be directed to achieve the goal with full cooperation between concerned parties at global, regional and national levels.

THE CHALLENGE OF THE PRESENT

HUMAN RESOURCES

The field survey carried out under the auspices of the Ministry of Health has covered 1,609 out of a total of 1,821 health centers (Table 5). By the time of the survey (mid 1985) the health centers were classified into four categories A 12%, B 22%, C 14%, and D 52%. Type A health center is the largest, usually staffed by more than one physician and several health assistants, whereas type D is the smallest and staffed by one physician and fewer health assistants. This classification has been abolished recently, however, a reference to the type of the health center will be made in the discussion.

Table 5 shows the distribution of the 1,609 health centers according to regions. Generally, the health centers serve small populations. In 51% of the cases a health center provides services for a population of 10,000 or less (Table 6). Of the total health centers surveyed, 77% were in rural areas where a health center provides services for an average of seven villages inhabited by a total population of 6,500 to 30,000 people. Some features of the health centers were studied, (Table 7). The majority of the health centers were easily accessible to the people and not far away from secondary health care. Two-thirds of the health centers were situated in rented houses, 49% were cleaned by contractors and 61% were provided with cars.

There were 22,732 persons working in the 1,609 health centers. Their distribution according to nationality and sex is shown in Table 8. Of the total there were 15,586 skilled persons (9.7 per health center) including physicians, dentists, pharmacists, health assistants, nurses and administrators. In addition there were 7,146 non-skilled persons (4.4 per health center). Table 9 shows the distribution of some categories of the health personnel according to regions.

Table 5. The Distribution of 1,609 Health Centers in Saudi Arabia According to Regions.

Region	Health Centers	
	No.	%
Central	287	17.8
Western	220	13.7
Eastern	211	13.1
Madinah	203	12.6
Asir	198	12.3
Baha	118	7.3
Qasim	113	7.0
Jizan	85	5.3
Northern	69	4.3
Hayil	67	4.2
Najran	38	2.4
Total	**1,609**	**100%**

Table 6. The Range of People Served by the Health Centers.

No. of People	No. of HC	%
- 10,000	818	50.8%
10,001 - 20,000	271	16.8%
20,001 - 30,000	172	10.7%
30,001 - 40,000	76	4.7%
40,001 - 50,000	88	5.5%
50,001 and over	184	11.5%
Total	**1,609**	**100%**

Table 7. Some Features of the Health Centers

Situated in governmental buildings*	34%
Provided with main electricity**	51%
Cleaned by a contractor+	49%
Accessible by asphalted road	64%
Provided with emergency car(s)	61%
Average distance from nearest hospital	46 km
Health centers within 10 km of a hospital	23%

* The rest were situated in rented house
** The rest were supplied by private generators
+ The rest were cleaned by employed janitors.

In a study of Qasim province[23] the physician in the health center examined about 90 patients per day spending about 2 minutes per patient. The services were predominantly curative. In Al Asiah Region, Qasim, ten health centers were evaluated and were found to be 'mostly curative' and to 'mainly treat sick people visiting the units'.[24]

The same pattern of curative services was observed in Khulais[25] and Tamnia[26] communities. According to a study sponsored by the Ministry of Planning[3] 'the health services available to the general population are predominantly oriented towards curative services. Mother and child care, antenatal care, information on proper dietary habits, prophylactic routine examinations of preschool children, etc. are insufficient.'

The deficiency in the health centers is a global phenomenon even in industrialized countries. Beales[27] in her study of health centers services in Britain wrote 'they (health centers) are meant to represent, encourage and facilitate progress, and by this criterion of their well-being most of them, in fact, are pretty sick.'

The unhealthy situation of health cneters is a repercussion of the hospital-based and curative-oriented medical education system prevailing today in the world.

THE PROMISES OF THE FUTURE

Recently the Ministry of Health has taken an important step towards improving the present situation. Several health centers are selected from different regions to be promoted from being curative oriented to become comprehensive primary health care centers. Also training courses are being held for health personnel to adopt the comprehensive health approach. Some regions such as Hail, Baha, Najran, Jizan and Qasim are making an impressive lead in the right direction.

The positive political commitment of primary health care is equally important. According to the Fourth Development Plan:[14] "The emphasis on health services provided through primary health centers will lead to an expansion in their responsibility for public health, health education and preventive health care programs. Vulnerable segments of the population, especially children, women and elderly citizens, continue to need basic health services. The public health programs in the Fourth Plan period aim to reduce infant and perinatal mortality and morbidity rates through greater control of infectious diseases, including the expansion of effective immunization activities."

However, the reorientation of a 'system' is a complex subject and needs to be carefully planned and directed. I will quote two examples of how plans for change were not fully carried out:

In 1978 a 10-day refresher course was held in Abha for 25 physicians working in health centers. The Objective was to orient them to the concepts and methods of comprehensive primary health care. They completed the course with fresh ideas on how they should improve their work. However, 6 months later they were found practicing the same way as they did before, viz: curative medicine. A change in practice needs more than an orientation course. It requires, in addition, a change in the working conditions, policies and regulations.

The second example comes from the Gwaiz health center in Jeddah. A decision was made to convert the curative oriented health center into a comprehensive primary health care center for a population of 15,000. More staff, money and facilities were injected into the center, but still the objectives were not achieved. No defined plan of action was drawn to meet specific targets. Only two physicians and a health visitor out of the 21 working staff had been through an orientation program of primary health care. The function of the health center was seen by the majority of the staff as to screen patients. 'We are the first point of contact for patients; we examine them, treat them and refer difficult cases to the hospital' said one of the physicians.

Comprehensive health care can never be achieved if the health personnel remain behind the walls of the health center and become occupied all the time by seeing and treating individual patients. The time of the staff should be divided between taking care of the out-patients and interacting with the whole community to prevent diseases and promote health. In order to free physicians from having to see all the out-patients, other members of the health team should be trained to treat simple cases which usually constitute 70% of the out-patients. Only the difficult cases need to be referred to the physicians who then will have the time to lead and supervise comprehensive health care.

The patients who attend the health centers constitute the tip of an iceberg (Fig. 4). Many people in the community, although looking healthy, are actually at risk and need care. For one reason or another they do not come to the health center. They include:

Mothers who need antenatal, neonatal and postnatal care, health education and nutritional programs, etc.

Children who need immunization, routine well-baby clinics, nutritional programs, dental hygiene, etc.

The elderly, convalescents and the disabled who need home care, nursing, rehabilitation programs, etc.

Figure 4. The iceberg pattern. The patients attending the health center are small in number compared to people at risk who do not attend the health center

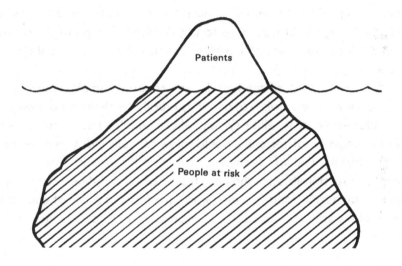

Drug addicts, the emotionally disturbed, the accident-prone and others who need help to change their lifestyle.

Unless the health team go beyond the walls of the health center to the community, they will never be able to explore and meet the actual needs of the population. Figure 5 shows two models of health centers, a curative oriented health center, and a comprehensive health center (a health center without walls).

Increasing the number of physicians does not solve the problem, not only because it is an expensive solution, but also because most physicians will spend their time carrying out simple tasks, less challenging and less productive than those they are prepared for.

Taylor[28] gave an interesting example of a role-reallocation from his experience in Narangual. 'A fascinating feature of the relocation of tasks was that much of the acute medical care that crowds doctor's offices, out-patient departments and hospital wards turned out to be routinizable and effectively delegated.' He trained auxiliaries to diagnose and treat dehydration, marasmus and pneumonia and to give nutritional supplements. The auxiliaries even extended their preventive care to homes. 'Within a year mothers were rehydrating infants on their own in their homes and diarrhea mortality had been cut by half... rehydration unit could be closed down because cases were cared for in the home... and mortality (from pneumonia) fell by half in a year'. In Saudi Arabia, ARAMCO medical services applied a successful program of screening patients by qualified nurses who proceeded to treat simple cases and to refer difficult ones to physicians.[29] This proves that Saudi patients will accept a health assistant or a nurse to attend to their minor ailments.

In our survey 51% of the health centers served small communities of 10,000 people or less (Table 6) and they usually functioned independently. As an alternative, a satellite system where smaller health centers come under the aegis of larger ones, would allow for consolidation of resources and decentralization of decisions. Each satellite should function as an integral unit responsible for the health services in a defined community. If adequate authorities and facilities were given and a sense of competition generated the satellites could work progressively to achieve their defined goals.

WHICH WAY FORWARD?

Before we come to specific recommendations, we should agree about general concepts:

1. Health development is an integral part of socioeconomic development.

Figure 5(A).   A curative health center

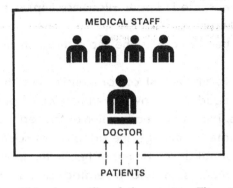

The function is within the walls of the center. The staff are inert and waiting for action.

Figure 5(B).   A comprehensive health center

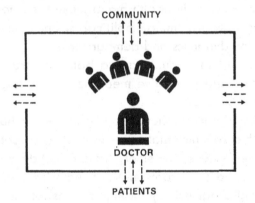

The function is within and out the center. The staff are active and health promoters.

2.   Factors such as housing, education, nutrition, safe water supply, and environmental sanitation contribute to the health of the people, even more than the health service *per se.*

3.   Multisectoral coordination is necessary to develop a comprehensive health services system.

4.   Health leaders, planners, educators and practicing physicians should realize that their responsibility is not only to cure illnesses but to maintain and promote health.

5. The population in general can be activated and trained to play a significant role in health planning, implementation, follow-up and evaluation.

6. Primary health care is the main thrust in the health services system.

7. In order to implement comprehensive health care there is an immense need to improve the utilization of physical and human resources. This entails reallocation of the health budget, the use of appropriate technology, the adoption of scientific management and above all development of health manpower.

8. Decision-makers in health-related sectors such as finance, planning, education, social welfare and municipalities need to be oriented to the objectives and to the functions of primary health care in order to gain their support.

9. Health executives and program directors should be provided with refresher courses in health management, economic budgeting, planning, programming, political science, human behavior, population dynamics and demography.

10. Medical students should have a balanced training in curative, preventive and promotive medicine. This is a great academic challenge by itself.

11. Practicing physicians should be oriented to the holistic approach to health care which makes a challenging career.

12. Family medicine is a re-emerging and fast developing specialty which gained solid roots in North America and Europe and is spreading progressively through the rest of the world. Training programs in family and community medicine in developing countries need thoughtful planning and direction to ensure their relevance otherwise they can easily become westernized.

Table 8. Personnel Working in 1,609 Health Centers According to Nationality and Sex.

| | Saudis | | Non-Saudis | | | | All Nationalities | | |
| | | | Arabs | | Non-Arabs | | | | |
	Male	Female	Male	Female	Male	Female	Male	Female	Total
Physicians (specialists)	15	3	578	103	225	70	818	176	994
Physicians (general)	23	15	1,573	300	728	160	2,324	475	2,799
Dentists	19	1	373	88	79	26	471	115	586
Pharmacists	8	3	199	9	40	2	247	14	261
Dietitians	6	—	6	6	2	—	14	6	20
Administrators	262	22	150	8	20	—	432	30	462
Nurses	560	180	1,139	1,975	549	2,349	2,248	4,504	6,752
Asst. pharmacist	140	—	252	41	678	36	1,070	77	1,147
Lab. technicians	83	—	359	89	338	133	780	222	1,002
X-ray technicians	39	—	155	21	192	41	386	62	448
Health inspectors	375	—	592	—	102	—	1,069	—	1,069
Asst. statisticians	18	7	13	7	1	—	32	14	46
Total skilled	1,548	231	5,389	2,647	2,954	2,817	9,891	5,695	15,586
Unskilled	4,667	973	508	67	813	118	5,988	1,158	7,146
Grand total	6,215	1,204	5,897	2,714	3,767	2,935	15,879	6,853	22,732

In every 10 health centers, there are, on average, 24 physicians, four dentists, 64 nurses and health assistants, two pharmacists, and three administrators (Table 10). A health center serves, on average, a community of 12,000 and is attended by 85 patients per day.

Health personnel in general and Saudis in particular are not attracted to work in health centers. Taking physicians for example, of 8,886 physicians working for the Ministry of Health, 65% are in hospitals, 34% in health centers and 1% in other units.

The Saudis constitute a minority of the staff in the health centers being 11.4% of the total skilled workers, 1.5% of the physicians, 3.4% of the dentists, 4.2% of the pharmacists, 11% of the nurses and 18% of the health assistants. Of the total 1,488 Saudi physicians working in the Kingdom only 56 work in the 1,609 health centers.

Many of the expatriates face cultural as well as language barriers (31% of the physicians and 43% of the nurses are non-Arab expatriates). These barriers are more deterrent in health centers than in hospitals since the contact with the community is more direct.

A high male to female ratio is the pattern among physicians (5 to 1), dentists (4 to 1), pharmacists (18 to 1), administrators (14 to 1), and health assistants (9 to 1), except nurses where the ratio is inverted (0.5 to 1).

The ratio of the total skilled to the non-skilled persons is (2.2 to 1) (Table 8). However, amongst the Saudis the ratio is inverted being (0.3 to 1). This reflects both, a general pattern among Saudi health personnel (a low ratio of skilled to non-skilled), and the preference of skilled Saudis to work in hospitals.

Of the total physicians working in the health centers 26% are specialists, many of whom hold diplomas requiring 2-3 years study in different specialties other than family medicine.

The question remains to what extent the health manpower resources are being utilized in order to promote the health of the people. The available data are not sufficient to make a judgment. In fact they raise more questions than they provide answers. There is an immense need for health services system researches and functional analysis studies in order to answer questions such as:

What is the most appropriate blend of sex and nationality for primary health care workers in a Saudi setting?

Table 9. Health Personnel Working in Health Centers Distributed According to Regions.

Region	No. of Health Centers	"All" Physicians	Dentists	Health Asst & Nurses	Total
Riyadh (Central)	287	758	117	2,086	2,961
Western	220	760	118	1,786	2,664
Eastern	211	610	92	1,667	2,369
Madinah	203	356	51	996	1,403
Asir	198	340	60	994	1,394
Baha	118	228	39	809	1,076

Qasim	113	265	41	828	1,134
Jizan	85	157	15	470	642
Northern	69	143	27	389	559
Hail	67	116	16	304	436
Najran	38	60	10	175	245
Total	**1,609**	**3,793**	**586**	**10,504**	**14,883**

How many physicians, public health nurses, health visitors, health educators, dietitians etc. do we need? How should they be prepared for their job and what function should they play?

How may family physicians do we need? How should they be trained and for what purpose?

Do the health educators need to be skilled professionals, trained front line health workers or a combination of both?

How and to what extent should the community be involved? What about native practitioners?

These and other questions should stimulate the search for the optimal team for primary health care in Saudi Arabia. All possible measures should be taken from now on to prepare Saudi health personnel for their future role in primary health care. No effort should be spared further to improve basic and continuing medical education and working and living conditions in rural areas.

By the year 2000 there will be 7,130 Saudi physicians (see p. 168). With their increasing number they will need to move to the periphery i.e. to the health centers. Another dimension is added to the situation in that by the year 2000 40% of the Saudi health workforce will be female.

Table 10. The Distribution of Skilled Personnel Working in 1,609 Health Centers.

	No.	Ratio Per Health Center
Physicians	3,793	2.4
Dentists	586	0.4
Pharmacists	261	0.2
*Health assistants	3,732	2.3
Nurses	6,752	4.1
Administrators	462	0.3
Total	**15,586**	**9.7**

* Health assistants include assistant pharmacists, laboratory technicians, X-ray technicians, statistical assistants, health inspectors, dietitians, etc.

THE PEOPLE

The people constitute a major health resource which is not yet fully tapped. They should participate in health planning, programming, implementation and evaluation. According to the Alma Ata resolution on primary health care 'community participation is the process by which individuals and families assume responsibility for their own health and welfare and for those of the community, and develop the capacity to contribute to their and the community's development.'[30]

In his opening address to the participants of an interregional seminar on primary health care, Dr H. Mahler, Director General of WHO said 'If they (people) are simply involved in the delivery of health care, without being actually involved in and identified with the management of primary health care, I can assure you that you are not getting the primary health care doctrine'[31]

From my personal experience in rural Saudi Arabia[32, 23, 25] people are always ready to participate if they are well informed of the objectives and the possible outcome of their involvement. It is part of the Islamic teaching 'Help ye one another in righteousness and piety, but help ye not one another in sin and rancour.'[33] Allah's Apostle Mohammad Ibn Abdullah carried the unburnt bricks to build the mosque in Madinah.

Table 7 shows that 66% of the health centers are located in rented buildings. Instead, people could be encouraged to provide the buildings freely for the health centers, an act which gives them a sense of self-reliance and in the meantime saves the rental costs. From the experience of a successful project in West Azerbaijan, Iran, it was found that if villagers are to identify with their health services, a health house should look as nearly like the other houses in the villages as possible.[18]

Paying nominal fees for services is another aspect of people participation. It also provides petty cash which could be used for the cleanliness and maintenance of the health centers. It could also help in cutting back some of the more unnecessary out-patients visits for social rather than medical reasons.

THE FUNCTION

Health centers are predominantly curative. Based on records from the last 4 months, 3.3 million people attended all 1,609 health centers in 1 month, an average daily attendance of 85 per health center. Table 11 shows a comparison of selected activities provided by two types of health centers (A and D) in 1 month. The numbers of deliveries and child vaccinations were quite low considering the average size of the communities (12,000 people). From the number of out-patients seen (an average of 85 per day), it is clear that preventive activities such as maternal and child health, health education and environmental sanitation were not effectively carried out. All patients were seen and treated by the physician himself who would have no time to lead or supervise other components of the health services.

In Turaba health center[32] two physicians were observed while working in the clinic. The average time spent by the physician taking care of a patient was 61 seconds and the performance was curative, or even palliative. 'The health center in Turaba has a minimum contribution to the promotion of health among the people.'[32]

Table 11. Selected Activities Carried Out by Health Centers A and D (average per month).

Activity	No. of Persons Who Received the Services	
	A	D
General out-patients	6,600	1,375
Dental patients	550	36
Radiological investigations	100	nil
Laboratory investigations	744	32
Minor surgery	21	6
Deliveries attended in the health center	5	1
Deliveries attended in the community	4	1
Children's BCG vaccination	22	3
Children's measles vaccination	30	5
Children's triple vaccination	53	10
Children's polio vaccination	55	10

In conclusion, primary health care concepts and methods should be appropriate to the Saudi setting and not imported from other cultures. The Alma Ata resolutions could be adopted with some modifications. Saudi

Arabia, although a developing country, has the unique feature of having a relatively high per capita income and scarce human resources. It is not impossible to find the right solution to its health problems but it will take time, effort and devotion.

HEALTH MANPOWER

During the last 15 years the number of physicians working in Saudi Arabia has increased 12 times, nurses nine times and health assistants six times[1] (Table 12).

In 1969 the first college of medicine and the college of pharmacy were inaugurated and by 1980 there were four colleges of medicine, and colleges of dentistry, pharmacy and health sciences, in addition to several postgraduate training programs. The college of medicine at the Gulf University, Bahrain has also been opened for Saudi students.

In this section the present situation and the future of selected categories of health personnel will be discussed. The discussion is meant to stimulate thinking rather than to give final judgements on such a complex subject.

THE CHALLENGE OF THE PRESENT

PHYSICIANS

In 1985, there were 14,335 physicians (78% males) working in Saudi Arabia, of whom 1,488 (10.4%) were Saudis (70% males) and the rest were expatriates mainly from Arab countries, India, Pakistan, Bangladesh, North America and Europe. Of the 1,488 Saudi physicians,

1,180 graduated from the colleges of medicine in Saudi Arabia and the rest graduated from abroad.

Table 13 shows the number of students and graduates from the colleges of medicine. Of the 1,413 graduates 1,290 (92%) were Saudis and the rest were from the Arab Gulf countries and North Yemen. Of the 2,865 students at present 15% are non-Saudis. Of the 1,290 graduates 1,180 work in Saudi Arabia and 110 are pursuing postgraduate training abroad.

Of the 220 physicians who graduated from the colleges of medicine in 1986, 40% were females. Medicine is one of the few available careers for females. Other choices are teaching, nursing, social welfare, pharmacy etc. but they are not as attractive to Saudi girls as a medical career. By the year 2000, it is estimated that women will constitute more than 40% of the entire Saudi medical workforce.

Saudi Arabia with its ratio of one physician to every 684 of the population, stands in a favorable position internationally. In the late 1970s there were 81 physicians for every 10,000 people in the world i.e. one physician for 1,235 people.[34] The range was from 1/520 to 1/17,000 according to the stage of

Table 12. The Number of Physicians, Nurses and Health Assistants Working in the Health Sector (Governmental and Private) 1970-1985.

Year	Physicians	Nurses	Health Assistants*
1970	1,172	3,261	1,741
1971	1,316	3,355	1,982
1972	1,704	4,370	2,230
1973	1,970	4,853	2,675
1974	2,641	5,857	3,215
1975	3,107	6,573	3,552
1976	3,734	7,839	4,208
1977	4,121	8,335	4,514
1978	4,612	8,728	4,823
1979	5,184	9,931	5,457
1980	6,536	12,133	6,642
1981	7,680	15,244	7,071
1982	8,663	16,965	8,226

1983	12,261	18,514	9,285
1984	12,971	22,781	11,058
1985	14,335	29,896	14,858

* Health Assistants: have, in general, 6-9 years of basic education plus 3 years of training in one of the following: radiology, anesthesia, laboratory, statistics, pharmacy, physiotherapy, etc.
From Ref. 1

Table 13. The Numbers of Medical Students and Graduates from the Colleges of Medicine.

College of Medicine at the University of:	No. of Students			No. of Graduates		
	Male	Female	Total	Male	Female	Total*
King Saud-Riyadh	763	485	1,248	480	189	669
King Saud-Abha	81	—	81	—	—	—
King Abdulaziz-Jeddah	438	411	849	286	227	513
King Faisal-Dammam	370	317	687	135	96	231
Total	**1,652**	**1,213**	**2,865**	**901**	**512**	**1,413**

* Of the 1,413 graduates, 1,290 were Saudis (92%). The rest were from the Arab Gulf countries and North Yemen.

development (Table 14). Many industrialized countries are facing today the problem of a surplus of physicians, and measures are being taken to limit the production of extra physicians and immigration of foreign doctors.[34] For example, of the 141,000 physicians in France 19,600 are unemployed — and this unhappy state of affairs is by no means confined to France.[35]

DENTISTS

The number of dentists working in Saudi Arabia is estimated at 1,200. The College of Dentistry, King Saud University (established in 1975) has produced 104 dentists and has 557 students enrolled (86% Saudis). With a yearly enrollment of 90 students (60 males and 30 females) at present which will increase to 150 by the year 1995, the total number of Saudi graduates by the year 2000 is estimated at 1,360. More Saudi dentists are still needed, and the establishment of another College of Dentistry is probably justified. The emphasis should be on the training of the dental health team with adequate orientation to dental hygiene.

Table 14. Health and Related Socioeconomic Indicators in the World.

Index	Least Developed Countries	Other Developing Countries	Developed Countries
Number of countries	31	89	37
Total population (millions)	283	3,001	1,131
Infant mortality rate (per 1000 live born)	160	94	19
Life expectancy (years)	45	60	72
% infants with birth weight of 2500 g or more	70%	83%	93%
% population with access of safe water supply	31%	41%	100%
Adult literacy rate	28%	55%	98%
GNP per capita	US$ 170	US$ 520	US$ 6,230
Per capita public expenditure on health	US$ 1.7	US$ 6.5	US$ 244
Public expenditure on health as % of GNP	1.0%	1.2%	3.9%
Population per doctor	17,000	2,700	520
Population per nurse	6,500	1,500	220
Population per health worker (any type including traditional birth attendant)	2,400	500	130

From *WHO Chron.* June 1981;35: 223.

Note: Figures in the table are weighted averages based on estimates for 1980 or for the latest year for which data are available.

PHARMACISTS

There are 3,253 pharmacists working in Saudi Arabia. From the College of Pharmacy, King Saud University (established in 1969) 636 pharmacists have graduated, of whom 363 were Saudis (57%). The first batch of 8 female pharmacists graduated in 1986. Of the 1,153 students enrolled in the college at present there are 687 Saudis (60%) with a male to female ratio of 1.4 to 1.

OTHER HEALTH PERSONNEL

In 1985 there were 44,754 allied health personnel of whom 29,896 were nurses and 14,858 were health assistants. Of the total 12% were Saudis. The Saudis are basically graduates from 17 health institutes for males (the first was established in 1959) and 15 health institutes for females (the first was established in 1961), all of them accept students after 9 years of basic education and train them for 3 years.

From the male health institutes 4,053 health assistants were graduated in various disciplines (Table 15) and there are 3,460 enrolled students. From the 15 female institutes 1,354 nurses were graduated and there are 1,038 enrolled students.

The training program for the allied health personnel faces some problems. There has always been a shortage of applicants especially females mainly because of the role model of a nurse or a health assistant is not popular. However, the situation has improved lately. In many instances office work is the path for promotion which drains technical persons to administrative jobs. Marriage frequently deters females from continuing their careers.

In 1978 the College of Allied Health was established in King Saud University. The 5-year bachelor degree program provides training in a variety of disciplines including rehabilitation, radiology, dental health, biomedical technology, community health and nursing. Since its establishment, only 26 males and 22 females had graduated. Saudis are not highly motivated to have medical technology for a career. Their training is only 2 years shorter than physicians and yet the socioenomic rewards are much less. Lately, the rate of employment has increased in the college because the doors were opened for the enrollment of non-Saudis. At present there are 947 students (636 males and 311 females) of whom only 35% are Saudis.

A bachelor degree program for allied health in King Abdul Aziz University in Jeddah has already produced 63 graduates of whom 85% were Saudis.

Table 15. The Graduates of the 17 Male Health Institutes up to 1986.

No.	Area of Training
809	Health inspectors
713	Nursing

400	Statistics
64	Nutrition
334	Anesthesia
336	Laboratory
366	Radiology
302	Operating theater
674	Pharmacy
55	Physiotherapy
4,053	**Total**

From the health institutes records.

POSTGRADUATE AND CONTINUING MEDICAL EDUCATION

Until recently postgraduate training was pursued only outside the country. In 1978 the Arab Board of Medical Specialties was established jointly by 16 Arab countries. Five specialties have already been approved; medicine, surgery, gynecology and obstetrics, pediatrics and family and community medicine. The training program lasts for 3-5 years and ends in the acquisition of a certificate which is highly regarded in the Arab world. Several training programs have started in Saudi Arabia jointly between the Universities, the Ministry of Health and other agencies such as the Ministry of Defense. In addition to the Arab Board, other postgraduate programs have been established in pediatrics, gynecology and obstetrics, opthalmology, psychiatry, primary health care, radiology, pathology and hospital administration leading to various diploma qualifications. King Faisal University in Dammam provides a 4 year postgraduate program in family and community medicine. At present there are 29 residents in the program and the first graduation will be in 1987.

The Joint Board for Postgraduate Medical Education was initiated in 1983 to promote and coordinate continuing medical education. The Board's membership includes: King Saud University College of Medicine, Riyadh Armed Forces Hospital, the Ministry of Health, the National Guard, the Security Forces Hospital and King Faisal Specialist Hospital and Research Center. The Board's activities include series of symposia and courses and examinations for foreign medical degrees (MRCP, FRCS, MRCOG, Canadian Evaluation Examination and FMGEMS).

The policy is to expand the postgraduate and continuing education programs to meet the apparent inclinations of Saudi medical professionals for specialization.

WHICH WAY FORWARD?

Several factors need to be considered in analyzing health manpower and planning for its development: the absolute and relative numbers of the health personnel, their knowledge, attitudes and skills, their geographic distribution, role allocations and the extent of their utilization. The prevailing health problems, the socioeconomic status of the population, the demographic pattern and the health needs and demands of the community also need to be considered.

A comprehensive analysis and plan for health manpower is beyond the scope of this book mainly because of the lack of sufficient data. However, based on the available data a pragmatic approach to the planning for the number of physicians required by the year 2000 will be presented. This is a preliminary discussion which is probably needed at this stage to stimulate critical thinking. A more scientific plan for the whole spectrum of health manpower, based on adequate information is very much needed.

A recent study[36] estimated the Saudi population at 7,042,149 in 1985 and 11,694,775 in the year 2000. The estimate was based on the results of the census conducted in 1974; which showed:

Total Population	7,012,000
Saudi Population	5,184,653
Natural growth rate	2.8% per annum

There is no available data on the number of expatriates, however, the total population (Saudi and non-Saudis) is estimated at 9.8 million in 1985 and 14 million by the year 2000. These estimates can be influenced by possible changes in birth rates, death rates and migration.

The future supply of the Saudi physicians can be estimated until the year 2000 with some degree of precision (Table 16). However, the establishment of a new college of medicine or a change in the enrolment policy would affect these predictions.

At present, the average yearly enrolment in the colleges of medicine is 155 students for Riyadh, Jeddah and Dammam colleges and 40 for Abha College. These numbers are expected to increase gradually within the next 10 years to 180 students for each of the first three colleges and 80 for Abha. In the period 1987-1991 there will be 2,191 Saudi graduates from the colleges of medicine in Saudi Arabia and 228 graduates from abroad. From 1992 to 2000, there will be 4,031 Saudi graduates from the four colleges of medicines in Saudi Arabia and 900 from abroad (mainly from Egypt, Bahrain, Europe, North America and Pakistan). The total number of Saudi physicians by the year 2000 is expected to be 7,130 after an allowance of 15% reduction due to death, retirement or change of career (Table 16). Emigration is not a significant factor in the foreseeable future.

In 1985 there were 14,335 physicians for a population of 9.8 million, a ratio of one physician to every 684 of the population which is similar to that in many industrialized countries (Table 14).

How many physicians are required for an estimated population of 14 million in the year 2000? This is a complex question and the answer is not easy, simply because there is no standard for the optimum ratio of physicians to population. The impact of health manpower on the health status of a population depends, besides the absolute and relative numbers of health manpower, on many variables as discussed above.

Until more information becomes available, a simple formula, the ratio of physicians to population, will be used to estimate the required number of physicians in Saudi Arabia by the year 2000. Arbitrarily three different ratios of physicians to population can be proposed.

Ratio of physicians to population	Number of physicians required
1:500	28,000
1:1000	14,000
1:1500	9,333

There could be a long debate on which ratio is most appropriate. I personally believe that if physicians, as members of the health team, are properly trained

Table 16. Number of Saudi Physicians 1986-2000.

Total students in the Medical colleges	2,865	
Students expected to be graduated by 1991 after an allowance of 10% drop out	2,578	
Saudi graduates by 1991 (85% of the total graduates)		2,191
Total physicians expected to be graduated 1992-2000 based on an average annual enrollment of 180 students in Riyadh, Jeddah and Dammam and 80 in Abha after an allowance of 15% drop out.	4,473	
Saudi graduates from 1992-2000 (85% of the total)		4.031
No. expected to be graduated from abroad 1987-2000.		1,128
Total Saudi graduates.		7,350
Saudi physicians available in 1985		1,488
Total you of Saudi physicians by the Year 2000 and after an allowance of 15% reduction due to death, retirement or change of career.		7,130

to meet the health needs of the country, properly distributed and properly utilized, a ratio of one physician to 1500 population could be more effective than a lower ratio with physicians not properly trained, distributed or utilized. For the sake of argument we will consider the 1:1000 ratio for the rest of the discussion.

For a population of 14 million in the year 2000 a total number of 14,000 physicians would be required. The expected Saudi physicians (7,130) will then constitute 51% of the total number required. The remaining 6,870 physicians will need to be recruited from abroad. They should be well selected and well prepared to understand the Saudi culture, the prevailing health problems and the best method of treatment and control, in order to contribute to the health development of the nation. Proper administration is always the cornerstone in a productive health service.

Other possible ways to cover the expected difference between the supply of indigenous physicians and the demand include:

1. Establishing a new College of Medicine. However, if the cost of establishing a fifth medical college was wisely spent on improving the quantity and quality of the members of the health team, it would probably be more beneficial.

2. Increasing the rate of admission to the existing four Colleges of Medicine might lead to a dilution of the educational resources.
3. Modifying the medical curricula by one or more methods.
    a. Reducing the years of training from 6 to 5. The dual objective of a medical college is to provide the graduate with the basics of medical knowledge, attitude and skills and to prepare him or her for a long life self-learning. Whether this could be achieved in 5 years is a matter of debate.
    b. Accepting suitable selected university graduates to study medicine for 3-4 years, a procedure which should save time and resources.
4. Selecting a ratio of one physician to 1200 population to be achieved by the year 2000 along with improving the role played by other members of the health team. Eyebrows will raise. A drop from a ratio of 1 to 684 in 1985 to a ratio of 1 to 1200 in the year 2000? The idea might look to be outrageous but nevertheless it deserves discussion.

CONCLUSION

The target of health services in Saudi Arabia is an integral part of the global target 'health for all by the year 2000.' It means the reduction of morbidity and mortality and the improvement of the health status of the population. The strategy to achieve the target does not need to be the most advanced or expensive, but rather the most appropriate. Health manpower development is the central theme in health services development and it requires:

Relating medical education to the health needs of the nation.
Better utilization of health manpower.
Establishing a School of Public Health.
Improving continuing medical education.
Studying, developing and controlling relevant aspects of traditional medicine.
Improving community reliance.

16. **Mahler H.** The meaning of health for all by the year 2000. *World Health Forum* 1981; 2: 5-22.

17. **Hellberg H.** Primary Health Care. *World Health Magazine* September 1983: 18-21.

18. **King M.** An Iranian experiment in primary health care: the West Azerbaijan Project. New York: Oxford University Press, 1983: 162-164.

19. **Fisek NH, Erdal Rengin.** Primary health care: a continuous effort. *World Health Forum* 1985; 6: 230-231.

20. **Habicht JP.** *Delivery of primary care by medical auxiliaries: techniques of use and analysis of benefits achieved in some rural villages in Guatemala.* Washington, PAHO, 1973. (PAHO Scientific Publication No. 278.)

21. *Progress in primary health care: a situation report.* Geneva: WHO Publication, 1983.

22. **Mahler H.** Health 2000: the monitoring process has been set in motion. *World Health Forum* 1984; 5: 99-102.

23. **Sebai ZA.** Primary health care in the district of Al Asiah. In: Sebai ZA, ed. *Community health in Saudi Arabia: a profile of two villages in Qasim region.* 2nd ed. Jeddah: Tihama Publications, 1984: 71-76.

24. **Banoub SN.** Primary health care in the Qasim region. In: Sebai ZA, ed. *Community health in Saudi Arabia: a profile of two villages in Qasim region.* 2nd ed. Jeddah: Tihama Publications, 1984: 59-70.

25. **Sebai ZA, Miller DL, Ba'aqeel H.** A study of three health centers in rural Saudi Arabia. *Saudi Med J* 1980; 1: 197-202.

26. **Sebai ZA, El-Hazmi MAF.** Health profile of preschool children in Tamnia villages, Saudi Arabia. *Saudi Med J* 1981; 2(Suppl 1): 68-71.

27. **Beales JG.** Sick health centres and how to make them better. Kent-London: Pitman Medical Publications, 1978: 137-147.

28. **Taylor CA.** Hospitals, primary care and health services research. In: *Proceedings of the role of hospitals in primary health care.* Karachi: Agha Khan Foundation 1981: 1-30.

29. **Oertley R, Hammer TS.** Saudi clinic design benefits patients flow, staff efficiency. *Modern Health Care* 1977; 7: 46-48.

30. *Alma-Ata 1978: Primary health care,* Report of the International Conference on primary health care, Alma Ata, USSR September

REFERENCES

1. *Achievements of the development plans (1970-1985).* Sc
    Arabia: Ministry of Planning, 1986; 271 pp.
2. *Kasongo Project Team.* Primary health care for less than a do|
    per year. World Health Forum 1984; 5: 211-215.
3. *Development of health services and its appropriate manpower (*
    Health Planner). Saudi Arabia: Ministry of Planning, 1984; 3
    pp.
4. **Sebai ZA, Miller DL, Ba'aqeel H.** A study of three health cente
    in rural Saudi Arabia. *Saudi Med J* 1980; 1: 197-202.
5. **Grants JB.** *Situation of children in the world.* UNICEF publicatio
    Oxford: Oxford University Press, 1986: 147-149. (Arabic)
6. *Statistics of children in UNICEF countries.* UNICEF Report. Ma
    1984:214-215.
7. **Girgis TH.** Health statistics advisory service in Saudi Arabia
    WHO Assignment Rep. EM/ST/125, EM/SAA/HST/001, 1983
    1-2.
8. **Sebai, ZA.** *The Health of the Family in a Changing Arabia: a case
    study of primary health care.* 3rd ed. Jeddah: Tihama Publications,
    1983: 117-128.
9. *World Health Statistical Annual.* Geneva: World Health
    Organization, 1985: 19-23.
10. **Grants JB.** *Situation of children in the world.* UNICEF publication.
    Oxford: Oxford University Press, 1985: 120-121. (Arabic)
11. **Searle CM, Gallagher EB.** Manpower issues in Saudi Arabia
    development. Milbank Memorial Fund Quarterly/Health and
    Society 1983; 61: 659-685.
12. **Sebai ZA.** *The health of the family in changing Arabia: a case
    study of primary health care.* 3rd ed. Jeddah: Tihama Publications,
    1983: 79-80.
13. **Serenius F, Fougerouse D.** *Health and nutritional status in rural
    Saudi Arabia.* **Saudi Med J** 1981; 2(Suppl 1): 10-22.
14. *Fourth Development Plan 1985-1990.* Saudi Arabia: Ministry of
    Planning, 1985: 323-338.
15. *International Conference on primary health care, Alma Ata,
    USSR, September 6-12, 1978. World Federation of Public Health
    Association,* Conference Bulletin 1978; 3: 1-2.

6-12, 1978. ("Health for all" series, No. 1) Geneva: World Health Organization, 1978: 50.

31. **Mahler H.** Opening Address. In: *Primary health care - the Chinese experience.* (Report of an Interregional Seminar) Geneva: World Health Organization 1983: 7-8.

32. **Sebai ZA.** *The health of the family in a changing Arabia: a case study of primary health care.* 3rd ed. Jeddah: Tihama Publications, 1983: 117-128.

33. *Kuran. Sura V; Maida* (The Table): 2.

34. **Fulop T, Roemer MI.** *International development of health manpower policy.* WHO Offset Publication No. 61, Geneva: WHO 1982; 149-162. (Arabic)

35. **Eraj YA.** Point of View: Too few doctors in the third world, too many elsewhere. *World Health Forum* 1985; 6: 146-149.

36. **Nutfaji MA.** *Projection of Saudi population by sex and age 1975-2000.* Saudi Arabia: Department of Mathematics and Financial Sciences, Research Center, College of Administrative Sciences, King Saud University 1981; 82 pp. (Arabic)

PROBLEM SOLVING EXERCISES

The following topics are meant to be teaching aids. It is anticipated that students will have read the appropriate portions of text beforehand. Then, having arrived in the class the students can discuss some of the topics listed below with the teacher adopting the role of moderator and commentator.

HEALTH PROBLEMS

Malaria

1. The malaria control program in Saudi Arabia.
2. The malaria situation in Saudi Arabia in the 1980s.
3. Oasis malaria.
4. The relationship between malaria and sickle cell disease.
5. Passive vs. active case detection.
6. Problems facing malaria control in Saudi Arabia.

Schistosomiasis

1. Global distribution of schistosomiasis.
2. The history of schistosomiasis in Saudi Arabia.
3. The natural history of the disease.

4. Clinical picture and possible complications.
5. Effect of ecological change on schistosomiasis.
6. The theory of disease dissemination in Saudi Arabia.
7. The magnitude of the problem in Saudi Arabia.
8. Schistosomiasis control program.
9. The future of schistosomiasis in Saudi Arabia.

Tuberculosis

1. Tuberculosis as a global problem.
2. Tuberculosis as a national problem.
3. The etiology, clinical picture and possible complications of gastrointestinal tuberculosis.
4. Treatment of pulmonary tuberculosis.
5. Measures to control tuberculosis in Saudi Arabia.
6. Problems involved in the control of tuberculosis in Saudi Arabia.
7. The future of tuberculosis in Saudi Arabia.

Viral Hepatitis (Type B)

1. Types of hepatitis.
2. Viral hepatitis (type B) as a global problem.
3. Immunology of viral hepatitis (type B).
4. Methods of the viral transmission.
5. The magnitude of the problem in Saudi Arabia.
6. The vaccine.
7. The future problem of viral hepatitis (type B) in Saudi Arabia.

Trachoma

1. The global situation of trachoma.
2. Etiology and contributing factors.
3. Historical background of the disease in Saudi Arabia.
4. The magnitude of the problem in the 1980s in Saudi Arabia.
5. Trachoma as a cause of blindness.
6. Method of investigation at community level.
7. Trachoma control program.
8. Community participation in the control of the disease.

Nutritional Disorders

1. The synergetic relationship between malnutrition and infectious diseases.
2. The use of anthropometric measurements in nutritional surveys.
3. The problem of rickets in Saudi Arabia.
4. The effect of dietary habits on health.
5. Causes of stunting and wasting among pre-school children.
6. The value of breast feeding.
7. How breast feeding could be promoted in Qatif oasis.
8. Predominant causes of anemia in Saudi Arabia.

Diabetes Mellitus

1. The etiology of diabetes mellitus.
2. The clinical picture and possible complications of diabetes mellitus.
3. The problem of diabetes mellitus in Saudi Arabia.
4. The distinctive features of diabetes mellitus in Saudi Arabia.
5. Investigating diabetes mellitus at the community level.
6. Measures to control diabetes mellitus.

Disorders of Hemoglobin Synthesis

1. Etiology of sickle cell disease.
2. Sickle cell disease as a global problem.
3. Sickle cell disease as a national problem.
4. The relationship between sickle cell disease and malaria.
5. The modified picture of sickle cell disease in Saudi Arabia.
6. Thalassemia in Saudi Arabia.
7. Glucose-6-phosphate dehydrogenase - deficiency in Saudi Arabia.
8. Measures to control haemoglobinopathies.

Cancer

1. Primary and secondary prevention.
2. The difference in the rank order between Taylor and El-Akkad studies (Table 3).

3. Cancer of the esophagus as a global and a national problem.
4. The etiology and pathology of hepatocellular carcinoma.
5. A program to control cancer of the breast.
6. Possible trends in lung cancer among Saudis.
7. Knowledge and attitude of Saudis towards cancer.
8. A national cancer registry program.

Road Traffic Injuries

1. Road injuries as a leading cause of death in Saudi Arabia.
2. The factors contributing to the problem.
3. A program to control road injuries in Saudi Arabia.
4. The socioeconomic impact of road injuries in Saudi Arabia.
5. Reducing case fatality rate.
6. Rehabilitation program.
7. Drugs and road injuries.
8. Management of road injuries at a primary health care level.
9. Promoting defensive driving.

HEALTH SERVICES

An Overview

1. The governmental health services are provided by the Ministry of Health and 10 other agencies. Discuss the advantages and disadvantages of such diversity of health resources.
2. Comment on the controversial issue of the GNP per capita and IMR as shown in Table 3.
3. Discuss centralization vs. decentralization of the health services, with reference to Figure 2.
4. What are the factors contributing to the curative orientation of the health services?
5. You are the only physician working in a health center attended by 100 patients per day. How would you plan for a reliable and useful information system?
6. What are the practical measures necessary to achieve the first objective of the national health plan "Strengthening Primary Care"?
7. Why does the health information system lag behind the health services?

Primary Health Care

1. Many developing countries suffer from an irrational use of health resources and inappropriate training of health personnel. Give examples and discuss the possible reasons and outcomes.
2. The text refers to vertical programs. Could there be horizontal and diagonal programs? Give examples. Discuss the advantages and disadvantages of each system.
3. Are you optimistic or pessimistic about the goal "Health for all in the year 2000"? Why?
4. An average health center in Saudi Arabia is staffed by a skilled health personnel, serves 1,200 people, is attended by 85 patients per day, and its function is predominantly curative. Draw a plan of action for such a health center in order to provide comprehensive health care. Do not hesitate to ask for additional resources or information if necessary. Be innovative and practical.
5. Health personnel in general, and Saudis in particular, are not attracted to work in health centers. As a Deputy Minister of Health how would you improve the situation?

Health Manpower

1. This is a subject for debate. Saudi Arabia has a ratio of one physician to 684 inhabitants. Considering the present situation and the predictable changes in the future, what would be the most appropriate ratio in the year 2000? Defend your argument.
2. Dental caries is a problem in Saudi Arabia. Discuss the possible etiology. How could the problem be solved?
3. Study the present situation of one of the Health Institutes and prepare a concise plan for its development.
4. Study the need for continuing medical education in a sample of health centers.
5. Elaborate on the basic information needed for the planning of health manpower development.
6. The Minister of Health assigns you the following problem to solve. "What is the most appropriate number and type of health personnel needed for an average comprehensive health care center in Saudi Arabia?" How would you deal with the task?

7.   How can the community be involved in the planning and management of primary health care?

8.   Table 1 shows selected activities carried out by health centers A & D in one month. Discuss.

9.   As a Deputy Minister of Health, how would you handle the situation of the primary health care physician who sees his patient in about two minutes?

10. This is a topic for debate. "In order to free PHC physicians from having to see all the outpatients, other members of the health team should be trained to treat simple cases." Do you agree or disagree? Defend your argument.

LIST OF TABLES

Trachoma

Nutritional Disorders

Cancer

Road Traffic Injuries

An Overview

LIST OF FIGURES

REFERENCES

Chapter I

HEALTH PROBLEMS

MALARIA:

1. **Doughty CM.** *Travels in Arabia deserta.* London: Jonathan Cape, 1921.
2. **Philby H, St. J.** *The Empty Quarter.* London: Methuen, 1933.
3. **Scott H.** *In the High Yemen.* London: Murray, 1942.
4. **Marett WC.** Some medical problems met in Saudi Arabia. *US Armed Forces Med J* 1953; 4: 31-38.
5. *Epidemiology Bulletin,* Dhahran, Saudi Arabia: Aramco Medical Department, Oct. 1972: 1-2.
6. **Daggy RH.** *Oasis malaria* (Third Conference of the Industrial Council of Tropical Health, Harvard School of Public Health). Industry and Tropical Health III 1957; 3: 49-56.
7. **Daggy RH.** Malaria in oases of eastern Saudi Arabia. *Am J Trop Med Hyg* 1959; 8: 223-291.
8. **Farid MA.** The implications of *Anopheles sergenti* for malaria eradication programmes east of the Mediterranean. *Bull WHO* 1956; 15: 821-827.

9. **Daggy RH.** Malariometric evidence of DDT resistance in *Anopheles stephensi* in cases of Eastern Saudi Arabia. In: *Proceedings of the Sixth International Congress of Tropical Medicine and Malaria.* Lisbon, Portugal, 1958.

10. *Epidemiology Bulletin,* Dhahran, Saudi Arabia: Aramco Medical Department, Nov 1974: 1-3.

11. **Gelpi AP.** Agriculture, malaria and human evolution. A study of genetic polymorphisms in the Saudi oasis population. *Saudi Med J* 1983; 4: 229-234.

12. *Malaria control program in the Kingdom of Saudi Arabia 1983.* Malaria Department, Ministry of Health, Riyadh, 1948: 9-28.

13. **Magzoub M.** *Plasmodium falciparum and Plasmodium vivax* infections in Saudi Arabia, with a note on the distribution of anopheline vectors. *J Trop Med Hyg* 1980; 83: 203-206.

14. *Intercountry malaria meetings of representatives from the Arab States of the Gulf Area.* Official report, Malaria Department, Ministry of Health, Riyadh, Oct 1977: 1-3.

15. *Report on malaria control program in the Kingdom of Saudi Arabia, 1979.* Malaria Department, Ministry of Health, Riyadh, 1980: 1-5.

16. *Malaria control program in the Kingdom of Saudi Arabia, 1983.* Malaria Department, Ministry of Health, Riyadh, 1984: 9-54.

17. **Carson RL.** *Silent spring.* Greenwich Conn Fawcett Publications 1962: pp. 304.

18. Anonymous. *Informal consultation of planning strategy for the prevention of pesticide poisoning.* Geneva: World Health Organization 1986, WHO/VBC/86.926: 28 pp.

19. **Farid MA.** *Malaria in Saudi Arabia.* Malaria Department, Ministry of Health, Riyadh, 1982: 16-19.

SCHISTOSOMIASIS:

1. **Mott KE.** Schistosomiasis - new goals. *Magazine WHO Dec.* 1984: 3-4.

2. **Hatch WK.** Bilharzia haematobium. *Lancet* 1887; 1: 875.

3. **Clemow FG.** *The geography of disease.* London: Cambridge University Press, 1903: 570 pp.

4. **Abdel Azim M, Gismann A.** Bilharziasis survey in south-western Asia. *Bull WHO* 1956; 14: 403-456.

5. **Tarizzo ML.** Schistosomiasis in Saudi Arabia. *Vemes. Congres Internationaux de Medecine Tropical et du Paludisme* (Excerpt) 1956.

6. **Tarizzo ML.** Schistosomiasis in Saudi Arabia: treatment with lucanthone hydrochloride (nilodin) and with sodium antimonyl gluconate (triostam). *Am J Trop Med Hyg* 1956; 6: 145-149.

7. **Farooq M.** Report on a visit to Saudi Arabia. WHO *Assignment Report* 1961; EM/BIL/19/SA24: 21 pp.

8. **Alio IS.** *Epidemiology of schistosomiasis in Saudi Arabia with emphasis on geographic distribution patterns.* Dhahran: Aramco, 1967. 217 pp. Dissertation.

9. **Arfaa F.** Studies on schistosomiasis in Saudi Arabia. *Am J Trop Med Hyg* 1976; 25 (2): 295-298.

10. **Davis A.** Schistosomiasis control in the Kingdom of Saudi Arabia with special reference to chemotherapy. WHO *Assignment Report* 1977.

11. **Habib MA, Morsy TA, El Nayal NA, Shoura MI.** Study of the clinical pattern of bilharziasis in Saudi Arabia. *J Egypt Soc Parasitol* 1977; 7: 163-170.

12. **Magzoub M, Kasim AA.** Schistosomiasis in Saudi Arabia. *Ann Trop Med Parasitol* 1980; 74 (5): 511-513.

13. **Wallace DM.** Urinary schistosomiasis in Saudi Arabia. *Ann R Coll Surg Eng* 1979; 61: 265-270.

14. **Gremillon DH, Geckler RW, Kuntz RE, Marraro RV.** Schistosomiasis in Saudi Arabian recruits, a morbidity study based on quantitative egg excretion. *Am J Trop Med Hyg* 1978; 27 (5): 924-927.

15. **Cutajar CL.** Urinary schistosomiasis in the Asir district of Saudi Arabia. In: Mahjoub ES ed. *Proceedings of the 5th Saudi Medical Meeting* Riyadh: College of Medicine, University of Riyadh, 1981: 543-552.

16. **Ibrahim AM, Sebai ZA,** Analytic study of patients attending the bilharzia clinic in Riyadh, Saudi Arabia. *SMJ* 1978; 16: 14-12.

17. **Hanash KA, Bissada NK, Abla A, Esmail D, Dowling A.** Predictive values of excretory urography, ultrasonography, computerized tomography, and liver and bone scan in the staging of bilharzial bladder cancer in Saudi Arabia. *Cancer* 1984; 54: 172-176.

18. **Arfaa F.** Schistosomiasis control in the Kingdom of Saudi Arabia. *WHO Assignment Report 1984;* EM/SCHIS/89-SAA/MPD/002.

19. **Arfaa F.** Schistosomiasis control programme in the Kingdom of Saudi Arabia. *WHO Assignment Report 1984;* EM/SCHIS/SAA/MPD/002.

20. **Githaiga HK.** *Fact finding visits to bilharzia centers in the Kingdom of Saudi Arabia.* Report to the Ministry of Health Department of Preventive Medicine - Bilharziasis Section 1984.

21. **Abdel-Wahab MF.** Changing pattern of schistosomiasis in Egypt 1935-79. *Lancet 1979;* 4: 242-4.

TUBERCULOSIS:

1. **Davidson PT.** Tuberculosis, new views of an old disease. *New Engl J Med 1985;* 312: 1514-1515.

2. Anonymous. *Sixth report on the world health situation 1973-1977* Part I: global analysis. (Arabic) Geneva: World Health Organization 1982: 112-114.

3. **Abrams JS, Holden WD.** Tuberculosis of the gastrointestinal tract. *Arch Surg 1964;* 89: 282-293.

4. **Papanikalaou B.** *The tuberculosis control program in Saudi Arabia.* WHO/TBC/10; 1949: 20-23.

5. **Sebai ZA.** *The health of the family in changing Arabia.* Jeddah: Tihama Publications, 1983: 93-95.

6. **Hammam HM, Kamel LM and Hidayat NM.** A health profile of a rural community in the Western Zone of Saudi Arabia. In: *Proceedings of the 4th Saudi Medical Conference.* Dammam: King Faisal University, 1980: 35-49.

7. **Grimes J, Sparrow JY, Woodbine A.** Program of health education and health screening in schools. *Saudi Child 1980;* 1: 22-28.

8. **Rowlands DF.** Tuberculosis sensitivity in a Saudi military school population. *Saudi Med J 1984;* 5: 183-189.

9. **Gultekin MS.** Tuberculosis control. *WHO Assignment Report* 1971, EM/TB/119. 25 pp.

10. **Aramco Medical Department.** Active pulmonary tuberculosis cases reported by Aramco health facilities, 1956-1976. *Epidemiol Bull 1976:* 1-3.

11. **The Ministry of Health, Kingdom of Saudi Arabia.** *Ann Rep* 1399H. (1979): 199-358.

12. **Shanks NJ, Khalifa I, Al Kalai D.** Tuberculosis in Saudi Arabia. *Saudi Med J* 1983; 4: 151-156.

13. **Rifai E.** *Tuberculosis in Arab countries.* Al Majallah Al Tibbiah Al Saudia (Arabic) 1982; 1: 86.

14. **Froude JRL, Kingston M.** Extra pulmonary tuberculosis in Saudi Arabia: a review of 162 cases. *King Faisal Specialist Hospital Med J* 1982; 2: 85-95.

15. **Salam KM, Bedeiwy AF, Saad A, Merdad.** In: *Proceedings of the 6th Saudi Medical Conference,* Jeddah: King Abdul Aziz University, 1981.

16. **Wazna MF.** Gastrointestinal tuberculosis. *King Abdul Aziz Med J* 1981; 1: 16-73.

17. **Lifeso RC.** Preliminary study of tuberculosis of the spine. *King Faisal Specialist Hospital Med J* 1982; 2: 3-13.

18. **Tongia RK, Fonseca V, Al-Nozha M, Fawzy ME.** Takayasu's disease in an Arab male: relationship with tuberculosis. *Saudi Med J* 1985; 6: 113-118.

19. **Gallen CS.** Assignment report, tuberculosis control, Saudi Arabia. WHO Regional Office for the Eastern Mediterranean, *Saudi Arabia* 1201 (Ex 0013) 1972; 1-8.

20. **Aneja KS.** Tuberculosis in Saudi Arabia: WHO *Assignment Rep* EM/TB/164-SAA/ESD/001. 1984: 3-4.

21. **Comstock GW.** Tuberculosis. In: Last JM (ed.) *Maxcy-Rosenau Public Health and Preventive Medicine.* 11th ed. New York: Appleton-Century-Crofts, 1980: 205-220.

VIRAL HEPATITIS:

1. **Jamjoom GA, Higham R.** Prevalence of viral hepatitis type B surface antigen (HBsAg) in patients with liver disease and in the general patient population at King Abdulaziz Hospital, Riyadh. In: Mahgoub E, ed. *Proceedings of the 5th Saudi Medical Meeting.* Riyadh: College of Medicine, University of Riyadh, 1980; 331-339.

2. **Moas A, Admaway AMO, Talukder MAS, Gilmore R.** Prevalence of hepatitis in the patient population of Riyadh Al-Kharj Hospitals Programme. In: *Proceedings of the 7th Saudi Medical Meeting.* Dammam: King Faisal University, 1982: 252-255.

3. **Talukder MAS, Gilmore R, Bacchus RA.** Prevalence of hepatitis B surface antigen among male Saudi Arabians. *J Infect Dis* 1982; 146: 446.

4. **Shafi MS, Mounsey G.** Prevalence of hepatitis B virus infection: experience at the National Guard King Khalid Hospital, Jeddah. In: Academic Committee ed *Abstracts of the 8th Saudi Medical Conference,* Riyadh: Saudi National Guard Medical Services Department 1983: 245.

5. **Maynard JE.** Hepatitis. In: Last **JM** ed. *Maxcy-Rosenau. Public Health and Preventive Medicine* 11th ed. New York: Appleton-Century-Crofts, 1980: 159-165.

6. **Basalamah AH, Serebour F, Kazim E.** Materno-Foetal transmission of hepatitis B in Saudi Arabia. *J Infect* 1984; 8: 200-204.

7. **Fathalla SE, Namnyak SS, Al-Jama AA** *et al.* The prevalence of hepatitis B surface antigen in healthy subjects residing in the Eastern Province of Saudi Arabia. *Saudi Med J* 1985; 6: 236-241.

8. **Sobeslavsky O.** Prevalence of markers of hepatitis B virus infection in various countries: A WHO collaborative study. *Bull Wld Hlth Org* 1980; 58: 621-623.

9. **Beasley RP, Hwang LY, Lin CC, Chien CS.** Hepatocellular carcinoma and hepatitis B virus: A Prospective Study of 22,707 Men in Taiwan. *Lancet* 1981; 1129-33.

10. **Peters RL.** Viral hepatitis: A Pathologic Spectrum. *Am J Med Sc* 1975; 270:17-31.

11. **Gelpi AP.** Fatal hepatitis in Saudi Arabian women. *Am J Gastrol* 1970; 53: 41-61.

12. **Gelpi AP.** Viral hepatitis complicating pregnancy: mortality trends in Saudi Arabia. *Int J Gyn Obs* 1979; 17: 73-77.

13. **Bhalerao VR, Desi VP, Pai DN.** Viral hepatitis in pregnancy. *Ind J Publ Hlth* 1974; 18: 165-70.

14. **Borha F. Haghighi P, Kekmat K, Rezaizadeh K.** Viral hepatitis during pregnancy: severity and effect on gestation. *Gastroentrology* 1973; 64: 304-312.

15. **Mallia C.** Hepatitis in pregnancy. *Br Med J* 1981; 283: 1546.

16. **Hilton PJ, Michael J, Wing AJ, Jones NF, Banatvala JE.** Hepatitis B virus and end-stage renal disease. *New Engl J Med* 1980; 303: 225-626.

17. **Shobokshi O, Serebour F.** Hepatitis B: problem in Saudi Arabia. In: Szmuness W. *et al.* eds. *Viral Hepatitis.* 1981 International Symposium. The Franklin Institute Press (Abstract) 673.
18. **Szmuness W.** Hepatitis B vaccine: demonstration of efficacy in a controlled clinical trial in a high risk population in the United States. *New Engl J Med* 1980; 303 (15): 833-841.
19. **Szmuness W, Stevens CE, Zang EA, Harley EJ, Kellner A.** A controlled clinical trial of the efficacy of the hepatitis B vaccine (Heptavax B): a final report. *Hepatology* 1981; 1: 377-385.
20. Hepatitis B virus vaccine safety: Report of an Interagency Group. *Morbid Mortal Wkly Rep* 1982; 31: 465.
21. **Abdurrahman MB.** Hepatitis B infection and immunization: A Review. *Saudi Med J* 1984; 5: 369-376.
22. **Little PJ.** Hepatitis B vaccination. *Saudi Med J* 1983; 4: 1-4.
23. **Larkworthy W.** Hepatitis B vaccination. *The King Faisal Specialist Hosp Med J* 1983; 3: 85-86.
24. **Haque K.** Hepatitis B vaccination. *Saudi Med J* 1983; 4: 275-276.
25. **Zuckerman AJ.** Priorities for immunization against hepatitis B. *Br Med J* 1982; 284: 686-688.

TRACHOMA:

1. **Majcuk J.** Trachoma control in the Eastern Mediterranean Region. *WHO Chron* 1976; 30: 97-100.
2. **Marret WC.** Some medical problems in Saudi Arabia. *US Armed Forces Med J 1953; 4: 31-38.*
3. **Page RC.** Progress report on the Aramco trachoma research programme. *Med Bull Standard Oil Co. (NJ)* 1959; 19: 68-73.
4. **Nichols RL** ed. *Trachoma research program: chlamydial research publications.* Dhahran, Saudi Arabia: Aramco/Boston, Massachusetts, USA: Harvard School of Public Health (1954-1981); 1982.
5. **Snyder JC, Page RC, Murray ES** *et al.* Observations on the etiology of trachoma. *Am J Opthalmol* 1959; 48: 325-329.
6. **Hanna AT.** *The epidemiology of trachoma and conjunctival infections in a Saudi Arabian oasis.* Harvard School of Public Health, Mass., USA: Department of Epidemiology. September, 1959. Doctoral thesis.

7. **Nichols RL, McComb DE, Snyder JC.** Chlamydia trachomatis infections of the eye in the Eastern Province of Saudi Arabia: a review of 21 years of research. In: *Proceedings of the 4th Saudi Medical Conference.* Dammam: King Faisal University, 1980: 77-103.

8. **Murray ES, Snyder JC, Bell SD Jr.** A note on the toxicity or white mice and gerbilles of a strain of elementary bodies isolated from a patient with trachoma in Eastern Saudi Arabia. In: *Proc 6th Int Congr Trop Med Malaria* 1958; 5: 530-535.

9. **Nichols RL, Von Fritzinger K, McComb DE,** Epidemiological data derived from immunotyping of 338 trachoma strains isolated from children in Saudi Arabia. In: Nichols RL (ed). *Trachoma and related disorders caused by chlamydial agents.* Amsterdam: Excerpta Medica, 1971; Series 223: 337-357.

10. **Nichols RL, Bobb AA, Haddad NA, McComb DE.** Immunofluorescence studies of the microbiological epidemiology of trachoma in Saudi Arabia. *Am J Opthalmol 1967; 63:* 1371-1442.

11. **Fenwick SA, McComb DE, Allen HF, Oertley RE, Nichols RL.** Catastrophic visual disabilities in Saudi Arabian villagers. Association of holoendemic trachoma, socio-economic factors and severity of disease sequellae, including blindness. (Submitted for publication).

12. **Mull JD, Peters JH, Nichols RL.** Immunoglobins, secretory component, and transferrin in eye secretions of infants in regions with and without endemic trachoma. *Infect Immun* 1970; 2: 489-494.

13. **Foster SO.** Trachoma in American Indian village. *Pub Hlth Rep* 1965; 80: 829-832.

14. **Taylor CE, Gulati PV, Harinarian J.** Eye infections in a Punjab village. *Am J Trop Med Hyg* 1958; 7: 42-50.

15. **Haddad NA.** Trachoma in Lebanon: observations on epidemiology in rural areas. *Am J Trop Med Hyg 1965; 14:* 652-653.

16. **Barenfanger J.** Studies on the role of the family unit in the transmission of trachoma. *Am J Trop Med Hyg* 1975; 24: 509-515.

17. **Attiah MAH, El Kholy AM, Omran AR.** Epedimiological pattern of initial trachoma infection in a rural community in UAR. *J Egypt Med Ass* 1962; 45: 623-637

18. **Nichols RL, Bell SD Jr., Haddad NA, Bobb AA.** Studies on trachoma: VI: microbiological observations in a field trial in Saudi Arabia of bivalent trachoma vaccine at three dosage levels. *Am J Trop Med Hyg* 1969; 18: 723-730.

19. **McComb DE, Nichols RL.** Antibodies to trachoma in eye secretions of Saudi Arab children. *Am J Epidemiol* 1969; 90: 278-284.

20. **Maitchouk I,** Epidemic haemorrhagic conjunctivitis pandemic of a new type of virus eye disease. *WHO/EM/VIR/4* 1972: 18 pp.

21. **Fletcher RJ, Voke J.** The need for eye correction training in Saudi Arabia. *Saudi Med J* 1982; 3: 119-123.

22. **Badr I, Qureshi I.** Ocular status of schoolchildren in Al Asiah Qasim Region. In: Sebai Z.A. ed. *Community health in Saudi Arabia: a profile of two villages in Qasim Region,* 2nd ed. Jeddah: Tihama Publications, 1984: 24-27.

23. **Badr I, Qureshi I.** Ocular status of school children in the town of Al-Majma'ah, Central Province, Saudi Arabia. *Saudi Med J* 1981; 2: 221-224.

24. Expert committee on trachoma (third report) World Health Organization. *Tech Rep Ser* 1962; 234: 15-19.

25. **Badr IA, Qureshi IH.** Cause of blindness in the Eastern Province of blind schools. *Saudi Med J* 1983; 4: 331-338.

26. **Tabbara KF, Badr IA.** Changing pattern of childhood blindness in Saudi Arabia. *Br J Ophthalmol* 1985; 69: 312-315.

27. **Tabbara KF, Badr IA, Paton D, Ross-Degnan D, Meaders R.** Survey of eye disease and blindness in the Kingdom of Saudi Arabia. *Opthalmology* 1984; 91: 141.

28. **Tabbara** KF. *Quarterly Report.* Research Department, Riyadh, Saudi Arabia: King Khalid Eye Specialist Hospital. 30th September 1984.

29. **Sebai Z.A.** Introduction to Qasim project. In: Sebai Z.A. ed. *Community Health in Saudi Arabia. A profile of two villages in Qasim Region,* 2nd ed. Jeddah: Tihama Publications, 1984: 1-10.

30. **Quran,** *Surat II Al-Bagara* (The Cow) verse 222.

31. **Quran,** *Surat V Al-Maaidah* (The Table) verse 6.

NUTRITIONAL DISORDERS:

1.   **Page RC.** Practical aspects of employee nutrition. *Indust and Trop Hlth* 1957; 3: 120-127.

2.   **Sebai ZA.** *The health of the family in a changing Arabia.* 3rd ed. Jeddah: Tihama Publications, 1983: 155 pp.

3.   **Sebai ZA, El Hazmi MAF, Serenius F.** Health profile of pre-school children in Tamnia villages, Saudi Arabia. In: *Priorities in Child Care. Saudi Med J* 1981; 2 (Suppl 1): 68-71.

4.   **Serenies F. Fougerouse D.** Health and nutritional status in rural Saudi Arabia. In: *Priorities in Child Care. Saudi Med J* 1981; 2 (Suppl 1): 10-22.

5.   **Hammam HM, Kamel LM, Hidayat NM.** A health profile of a rural community in the western zone of Saudi Arabia. In: *Proceedings of the 4th Saudi Medical Conference.* Dammam: King Faisal University, 1980: 26-34.

6.   **Abdulla MA, Sebai ZA, Swailem AR.** Health and nutritional status of preschool children. In: Sebai ZA. ed. *Community Health in Saudi Arabia: a profile of two villages in Qasim Region. Saudi Med J,* Monogr No. 1 2nd ed Jeddah: Tihama Publications, 1985: 11-18.

7.   **Wirths W, Hamdan M, Hayati M, Rajhi H.** Ernahrungsstatus, nahrungsverbrauch und nahrstoffzufuhr von schulern in Saudi Arabien: Anthropometriche Daten. *Zeitshrift fur Ernahrungswissenschaft* 1977; 16:1-11.

8.   **Humeida AK, Hardy MJ.** Birth weights, occipito-frontal circumferences and crown to heel lenghts in four-hundred normal, healthy Saudi Babies. In: Mahjoub ES, et al. eds. *Proceedings of the 5th Saudi Medical Meeting.* Riyadh: University of Riyadh, 1981: 419-427.

9.   **Laurance BM.** What can be done to keep Saudi children healthy? *Saudi Med J* 1982; 3: 221-224.

10.   **Hassan MM.** Multiple nutritional deficiencies and multiple infections. *King Abdulaziz Med J* 1982; 2: 51-58.

11.   **Mohamed AE, Madkour MM.** Pernicious anemia in a Saudi male. *Saudi Med J* 1984; 5: 201-203.

12.   **McNiel JR.** Variation in the response of childhood iron deficiency anemia to oral iron. *Blood* 1968; 31: 641-646.

13. **Sejeny SA, Khurshid M, Kamil A, Khan FA.** Anemia survey in the southwestern region of Saudi Arabia. In: *Proceedings of the 4th Saudi Medical Conference,* Dammam: King Faisal University 1980: 124-128.

14. **Hafez A. Marshall I.** A survey of anemia from June 1981 to January 1982 in the Department of Primary Care, Riyadh Al-Kharj Hospital Programme. In: *Proceedings of the 7th Saudi Medical Meeting,* Dammam: King Faisal University, 503-505.

15. **Fry J.** *Common diseases - their natural incidence and care.* 2nd edition Lancaster MTP Press Ltd, 1979: 209.

16. **Smart Sm, Duncan ME, Kalina JM.** Haemoglobin levels and anemia in pregnant Saudi women. *Saudi Med J* 1983; 4: 263-268.

17. **Hartley DRW.** One thousand obstetric deliveries in the Asir Province, Kingdom of Saudi Arabia: A Review. *Saudi Med J* 1980; 1: 187-196.

18. **Elidrissy ATH, Taha SA.** Rickets in Riyadh. In: Mahgoub ES, *et al.* eds. *Proceedings of the 5th Saudi Medical Meeting.* Riyadh: University of Riyadh, 1981: 409-418.

19. **Sedrani SH.** Low 25-hydroxyvitamin D and normal serum calcium concentration in Saudi Arabia: Riyadh Region. *Ann Nutrit Metab* 1984; 28: 181-185.

20. **Sedrani SH, Elidrissy ATH, El Arabi KM.** Sunlight and vitamin D status in normal Saudi subjects. *Am J Clin Nutr* 1983; 38: 129-132.

21. **Elidrissy ATH, El Swailem AR, Belton NR, Aldress AZ, Forfar JO.** 25-hydroxy vitamin D in rachitic, non-rachitic and marasmus children in Saudi Arabia. In: *Vitamin D, chemical, biochemical and clinical endocrinology of calcium metabolism.* Berlin-New York: Walter de Gruyter & Co, 1982: 617-619.

22. Anonymous. Medical, nutritional and social study of sample of Riyadh schoolgirls Department of Nutrition, Ministry of Health-1977: (Arabic).

23. Anonymous. Results of a field survey on health, nutrition and social welfare of preschool children in Riyadh, Department of Nutrition, Ministry of Health 1981: (Arabic).

24. **Sebai ZA, Shalaby EME.** The family setting. In: Sebai ZA. ed. *Community health in Saudi Arabia: a profile of two villages in*

Qasim Region. Saudi Med J, Monog No. 1, 2nd ed. Jeddah: Tihama Publications, 1985; 35-40.

25. **Lawson M.** Infant feeding Habits in Riyadh. In: *Priorities in Child Care. Saudi Med J* 1981; 2 (Suppl 1): 26-29.

26. **Elias JBT.** A survey of place of delivery, modes of milk feeding and immunization in a primary health care centre in Saudi Arabia. *Saudi Med J* 1985; 6: 169-176.

27. **Rahman J, Farrag OA, Chatterjee TK, Rahman MS, Al-Awdah S.** Pattern of infant feeding in the Eastern Province of Saudi Arabia. In: *Proceedings of the 7th Saudi Medical Meeting.* Dammam: King Faisal University, Dammam, 1982; 407-411.

28. **Hamidi E.** A call for clinical dietetic training in the Kingdom of Saudi Arabia. *Saudi Med J* 1981; 2: 44-47.

DIABETES:

1. **Cahill GF Jr.** Current concepts of diabetes. In: Marble A, Krall LP, Bradley RF, *et al.* eds. *Joslin's diabetes mellitus,* 12th edn. Philadelphia: Lea & Febiger, 1985; 1-11.

2. **Papper S.** Internal medicine. In: Frohlich ED ed. *Rypins' medical licensure examinations,* Philadelphia: JB Lipincott, 1981; 728-729.

3. **Berkow R,** ed. Diabetes mellitus. In: *Merk manual of diagnosis and therapy.* 14th edn. Rahway, New Jersey, USA: Merk & Co. Inc., 1982; 1037-1052.

4. **Scrimshow NS, Wray JD.** Nutrition and preventive medicine. In: Last JM, ed. *Maxcy-Rosenau public health and preventive medicine,* 11th edn. New York: Appleton-Century-Crofts, 1980; 1469-1503.

5. **Krolewski AS, Warram JH.** In: Marble A, Krall LP, Bradley RF, *et al.,* eds. *Joslin's diabetes mellitus,* 12th edn. Philadelphia: Lea & Febiger, 1985; 12-42.

6. **WHO Expert Committee on Diabetes Mellitus.** Technical Report Series 646. Geneva, World Health Organization 1980.

7. **Zimmet P.** Type 2 (noninsulin dependent) Diabetes. An epidemiologic overview. *Daibetologia* 1982; 22: 399-411.

8. **Neel JV.** Diabetes mellitus. A "Thrifty" genotype rendered detrimental by progress. *Am J Hum Genet* 1962; 14: 353-362.

9. **Bell JL, Chang P.** Glycosuria and diabetes mellitus in Saudi Arabia. *Saudi Med J* 1982; 3: 284-290.

10. **Bacchus RA, Bell JL, Madkour M. Kilshaw B.** The prevalence of diabetes mellitus in male Saudi Arabs. Diabetologia 1982; 23: 330-332.

11. **Bell JL, Bacchus RA, Madkour MM, Kilshaw BH.** The prevalence of diabetes mellitus in male and female Saudi Arabs. In: Bejaj JS *et al.* eds. *Diabetes mellitus in developing countries.* New Delhi Interprint 1984; 35-38.

12. **Bell JL, Bacchus RA.** Glucose tolerance in Saudi Arabs in relation to the criteria of the World Health Organization. *Saudi Med J* 1984; 5: 61-64.

13. **Bacchus R, Bell J.** Diabetes in Saudi Arabia. Hospimedica 1985; 9: 6-11.

14. **Kassimi MA, Khan MA.** Maturity onset diabetes of youth in Saudi patients: Is it a common problem? *Saudi Med J* 1981; 2: 146-148.

15. **Mathew PM, Hamdan JA.** *Presenting features and prevalence of juvenile diabetes mellitus in Saudi Arab children,* Aramco, Dhahran, Saudi Arabia: Pediat Service Division, 1982: 7 pp.

16. **Kyllo CJ, Nuttall FQ.** Prevalence of diabetes mellitus in school-age children in Minnesota. *Diabetes* 1978; 27: 57-60.

17. **Sterkey G, Holmgren G, Gustavson KH,** *et al.* The incidence of diabetes in Swedish children, 1970-1975. *Acta Pediat Scand* 1978; 67: 139-143.

18. **Joner G, Sovik O.** Incidence, age at onset and seasonal variation of diabetes mellitus in Norwegian children, 1973-1977. *Acta Pediat Scand* 1981; 70: 329-335.

19. **Lestradet H, Besse J.** Prevalence and incidence of diabetes mellitus in children and adolescents. *Acta Pediat Belg* 1977; 30: 123-124.

20. **Kingston M, Skoog WC.** Diabetes in Saudi Arabia. *Saudi Med J* 1986; 7: 130-142.

21. Abstracts. *Symposium on diabetes mellitus in Saudi Arabia* held on 4-5 May 1986 at Medical City King Fahd National Guard Hospital, Riyadh. The Joint Board of Postgraduate Medical Education, King Saud University, Riyadh. 1986: 34 pp. (Abstracts).

DISORDERS OF HEMOGLOBIN SYNTHESIS:

1. **Neel JV.** The inheritance of sickle cell anemia, *Science* 1949; 110: 64-66.
2. **Pauling L, Itano HA, Singer SJ, Well IC.** Sickle cell anemia, a molecular disease, *Science* 1949; 110: 543-548.
3. **Walters JH.** The tropical anemias. In: Wilcocks and Manson-Bahr, eds. *Mansons' tropical disease.* London: Bailliere Tindall, 1972: 21-37.
4. **El-Hazmi MAF.** The red cell genetics and environmental interactions - a Tehamat-Aseer profile. *Saudi Med J* 1985; 6: 101-112.
5. **Daggy RH.** Malaria in oases of Eastern Saudi Arabia. II, *Am J Trop Med Hyg* 1959; 8: 223-291.
6. **Gelpi AP.** Sickle cell disease in Saudi Arabia. *Acta Haematol* 1970; 43: 89-99.
7. **McNiel JR.** Family studies of thalassemia in Arabia. *Am J Hum Genet* 1967; 19: 100-111.
8. **Marajian G, Ikin EW, Mourant AE, Lehmann H.** The blood groups and haemoglobins of the Saudi Arabians. *Hum Biol* 1966; 38: 394-420.
9. **Lehmann H, Marajian G, Mourant AE.** Distribution of sickle cell haemoglobin in Saudi Arabia. *Nature* 1963; 198: 492-493.
10. **Gelpi AP.** Benign sickle cell disease in Saudi Arabia: survival estimate and population dynamics. *Clin Genet* 1979; 15: 307-310.
11. **Perrine RP, John P, Pembrey M, Perrine S.** Sickle cell disease in Saudi Arabs in early childhood. *Arch Dis Child* 1981; 56: 187-192.
12. **El-Hazmi MAF, Lehmann H.** Haemoglobin Riyadh - A2B2(120(GH3) Lys-Asn). A new variant found in association with a-thalassemia: and iron deficiency. *Haemoglobin* 1976; 1: 59-74.
13. **Perrine RP, Pembrey ME, John P, Perrine S, Shoup F.** Natural history of sickle cell anaemia in Saudi Arabia. *Ann Int Med* 1978; 88: 1-6.
14. **Pembrey ME, Wood WG, Weatherall DJ, Perrine RP.** Foetal hemoglobin production and the sickle gene in the oases of Eastern Saudi Arabia. *Br J Haematol* 1978; 40: 415-429.

15. **Pembrey ME, Perrine RP, Wood WG, Weatherall DJ.** Sickle-β-thalassemia in Eastern Saudi Arabia. *Am J Hum Genet* 1980; 32: 26-41.

16. **Bertles JF, Rabinovitz R, Dobler J.** Haemoglobin interaction; modification of solid phase composition in the sickling phenomenon. *Science* 1970; 169: 375-378.

17. **Pasvol G, Weatherall DJ, Wilson RJM.** Effects of foetal haemoglobin on susceptibility of red cells to plasmodium falciparum. *Nature* 1977; 270: 171-173.

18. **Pasvol G. Weatherall DJ, Wilson RJM.** Cellular mechanism for the protective effect of haemoglobin S against P. falciparum malaria. *Nature* 1978; 247: 701-703.

19. **Roth EF, Friedman M, Ueda Y, Tellez I, Trager W, Nagel RL.** Sickling rates of human AS red cells infected in vitro with Plasmodium falciparum malaria. *Science* 1978; 202: 650-652.

20. **Gelpi AP.** Migrant populations and the diffusion of the sickle-cell gene. *Ann Int Med* 1973; 79: 258-264.

21. **Weatherall DJ, Clegg JB.** *The thalassemia syndromes.* 2d ed. Oxford: Blackwell, 1972.

22. **Weatherall DJ.** Abnormal haemoglobins in the neonatal period and their relationship to thalassemia. *Br J Haematol* 1963; 9: 265.

23. **Pembrey ME, Weatherall DJ, Clegg JB, Bunch C, Perrine RP.** Haemoglobin Bart's in Saudi Arabia. *Br J Haematol* 1975; 29: 221-234.

24. **McNiel JR.** Family studies of alpha-thalassemia and hemoglobin H disease in Eastern Saudi Arabia. *J Med Assoc Thai* 1971; 54: 153-166.

25. **Pressley L, Higgs DR, Clegg JB, Perrine RP, Pembrey ME, Weatherall DJ.** A new genetic basis for hemoglobin-H disease. *New Engl J Med* 1980; 3: 1383-1388.

26. **Perrine RP, Pembrey ME, John P, Perrine S, Shoup F.** Natural history of sickle cell anemia in Saudi Arabia. *Ann Int Med* 1978; 88: 1-6.

27. **Gelpi AP.** Glucose-6-phosphate dehydrogenase deficiency in Saudi Arabia. *Blood* 1965; 25: 486-493.

28. **Bayoumi RA, Omer A, Samuel APW, Saha N, Sebai ZA, Sabaa HMA.** Haemoglobin and erythrocytic glucose-6-phosphate

dehydrogenase variants among selected tribes in Western Saudi Arabia. *Trop Geog Med* 1979; 31: 245-252.

29. **Gelpi AP, King MC.** New data on glucose-6-phosphate dehydrogenase deficiency in Saudi Arabia. *Hum Hered* 1977; 27: 285-291.

30. **Gelpi AP.** Glucose-6-phosphate dehydrogenase deficiency, the sickling trait, and malaria in Saudi Arab children. *J Pediat* 1967; 71: 138-146.

31. **Gelpi AP.** Glucose-6-phosphate dehydrogenase deficiency in Saudi Arabia. *Bull WHO* 1967; 37: 539-546.

32. **Lewis RA, Hathorn M.** Correlation of S hemoglobin with glucose-6-phosphate dehydrogenase deficiency and its significance. *Blood* 1965; 26: 176-180.

33. **El-Hazmi MAF, Warsy AS.** Aspects of sickle cell gene in Saudi Arabia - interaction with glucose-6-phosphate dehydrogenase deficiency. *Hum Genet* 1984; 68: 320-323.

34. **Gelpi AP.** Glucose-6-phosphate dehydrogenase deficiency: the sickling trait, and malaria in Saudi Arab children. *J Pediat* 1967; 71: 138-146.

35. **El-Hazmi MAF.** Haemoglobin disorders: a pattern for thalassaemia and haemoglobinopathies in Arabia. *Acta Haematol* 1982; 68: 43-51.

36. **Kandil OF, Saleh AA, Khater RA, Mohammed AM, Hindawy DS.** The course and outcome of pregnancy in Saudi females with sickle cell anaemia and sickle cell trait. In: *Proceedings of the 7th Saudi Medical Meeting.* Dammam: King Faisal University, 1982: 360-365.

37. **Al-Awamy B, Pearson HA, Wilson WA, Naeem MA.** Function of the spleen in Saudi patients with sickle cell anaemia. In: *Proceedings of the 7th Saudi Medical Meeting.* Dammam: King Faisal University, 1982: 439-445.

38. **El-Hazmi MAF.** Incidence and frequency of haemoglobinopathies and thalassaemia in the North-West sector of Arabia. *Saudi Med J* 1985; 6: 149-162.

39. **Hartley DRW.** One thousand obstetric deliveries in the Asir Province, Kingdom of Saudi Arabia: a review. *Saudi Med J* 1980; 1: 187-196.

40. **El-Hazmi MAF, Sebai ZA.** Laboratory tests profile for pre-school children at Tamnia (Aseer Province). *Saudi Med J* 1981; 2: 198-202.

41. **Lehmann H. Maranijan G, Mourant AE.** *Nature,* Lond 1963; 198-492.

42. **El-Hazmi MAF.** Human haemoglobin and haemoglobinopathies in the Arabian Peninsula - studies at the molecular level. In: *Proceedings of the 4th Saudi Medical Conference.* Dammam: King Faisal University, 1980; 317-324.

43. **Greenberg MS, Kass EH, Castle WB.** Studies in the destruction of red cells. XII. Factors influencing the role of S haemoglobin in the pathologic physiology of sickle-cell anemia and related disorders. *J Clin Invest* 1957; 36: 833-847.

44. **Wishner BC, Ward KB, Lattman EE, Love WE.** Crystal structure of sickle cell deoxyhaemoglobin at 5 A° resolution. *J Mol Biol* 1975; 98: 179-194.

45. **El-Hazmi MAF, Lehmann H.** Human haemoglobins and haemoglobinopathies in Arabia: Hb O Arab in Saudi Arabia. *Acta Haematol* 1980; 63: 268-273.

46. **Gelpi AP, King MC.** Screening for abnormal hemoglobins in the Middle East: new data on hemoglobin S and the presence of hemoglobin C in Saudi Arabia. *Acta Haematol* 1976; 56: 334-337.

47. **Brewer GJ, Brewer LF, Prasad AS.** Suppression of irreversibly sickled erythrocytes by zinc therapy in sickle cell anemia. *J Lab Clin Med* 1977; 90: 549-554.

48. **Brewer GJ, Bereza U.** Membrane therapy of sickle cell anemia with zinc and other drugs. In: Fried W, ed. *Comparative clinical aspects of sickle cell disease.* New York, Elsevier/North Holland, 1982: 175-187.

49. **Warsy AS, El-Hazmi MAF, Bahakim HM.** Molecular therapy of sickle cell anaemia - the state of the art. *Saudi Med J* 1985; 6: 257-263.

CANCER:

1. **El-Akkad SM, Amer MH, Lin GS, Sabbah RS, Godwin JT.** Pattern of cancer in Saudi Arabs referred to King Faisal Specialist Hospital. *Cancer* 1986 (in press).

2. **Taylor JW.** Cancer in Saudi Arabia. *Cancer* 1963; 16: 1530-1536.

3. **Azar HA.** Cancer in Lebanon and the Near East. *Cancer* 1962; 15:66-78.

4. **Perrine RP, Juma'a A.** Changing trends in cancer in Saudi Arabia. *Epedimiology Bulletin.* Dhahran: Aramco Medical Department, January 1975: 1-4.

5. **Gelpi AP.** Malignant lymphoma in Saudi Arabia. *Cancer* 1970; 25:892-895.

6. **Stirling G, Khalil AM, Nada GN, Saad AA, Raheem MA.** Malignant neoplasm in Saudi Arabia. *Cancer* 1979; 44: 1543-1548.

7. **Stirling GA, Khalil AM, Nada GM, Saad AA, Raheem MA.** A study of one thousand consecutive malignant neoplasms in Saudis 1975-1977. *Saudi Med J* 1979; 1: 89-94.

8. **Bin Ahmed OS, Sabbah RS.** Childhood non-Hodgkin's lymphoma in Saudi Arabia: Clinical features of 100 cases. *King Faisal Specialist Hosp Med J* 1982; 2: 217-224.

9. **Frazer JW.** Malignant lymphomas of the gastrointestinal tract. *Surg Gynec Obstet* 1959; 108: 182-190.

10. **El-Gazayerli M, Kharadly M, Khalil H, Galal R, Raid W, El-Gazayerli MM.** Primary tumors of lymph nodes. In: *Lymphoreticular tumors in Africa* (Symposium). Basel/New York: S. Karger, 1964: 36-41.

11. **Froede RC, Mason JK.** Malignant disease of Aden Arabs. *Cancer* 1965; 18: 1175-1179.

12. **Racoveanu NT.** Cancer activities in WHO Eastern Mediterranean Region during 1976. In: *WHO Second Meeting of the Regional Advisory Panel on Cancer*, Tunis, 18 Nov 1976; Annex IV: 1-7. v.

13. **American Cancer Society:** Cancer statistics, 1985. *Ca-A Cancer J Clinicians* 1985; 35: 19-35.

14. **El-Akkad S.** Cancer in Saudi Arabia: a comparative study. *Saudi Med J* 1983; 4: 156-164.

15. **Amer MH.** Pattern of cancer in Saudi Arabia: A personal experience based on the management of 1,000 patients, Part I. *King Faisal Specialist Hosp Med J* 1982; 2: 203-215.

16. **Koriech OM, Al Kuhaymi R.** Cancer in Saudi Arabia: Riyadh Al-Kharj Hospital Programme Experience. *Saudi Med J* 1984; 5: 217-233.

17. **Aur RJA, Sackey K, Sabbah RS,** et al. Combination therapy for childhood acute lymphocytic leukemia. *King Faisal Specialist Hosp Med J* 1985; 5: 79-89.

18. **Waterhouse JAH.** International epidemiology of cancer. *J R Coll Physicians Lond* 1985; 19: 10-12.

19. **Tuyns AJ, Pequignot G, Jenson DM.** Role of diet, alcohol and tobacco in esophageal cancer, as illustrated by two contrasting high-incidence areas in the north of Iran and west of France. *Front Gastrointest Res* 1979; 4: 101-110.

20. **Doll R.** Geographical variation in cancer incidence: a clue to causation. *World J Surg* 1978; 2: 595-602.

21. **Coordinating Group for the Research of Esophageal Carcinoma.** The epidemiology of esophageal cancer in north China and preliminary results in the investigation of its etiological factors. *Chin Med J* 1975; 1: 167-183.

22. **Mellow MH, Layne EA, Lipman TO et al.** Plasma zinc and vitamin A in human squamous carcinoma of the esophagus. *Cancer* 1983: 51: 1615-1620.

23. **Miller RW.** Cancer epidemics in the People's Republic of China. *J Natl Cancer Inst* 1978; 60: 1195-1203.

24. **Munoz N, Grassi A. Qiong S, et al.** Pre-cursor lesions of oesophageal cancer in high-risk populations in Iran and China. *Lancet* 1982; 1: 876-879.

25. **Van Rensburg SJ.** Epidemiologic and dietary evidence for a specific nutritional predisposition to esophageal cancer. *J Natl Cancer Inst* 1981; 67: 243-251.

26. **Al-Karawi M, Al Otaibi R, Kilbane AJ, Yassawy I.** High prevalence of oesophageal carcinoma - results of three-year retrospective study of 1,550 upper gastro-intestinal endoscopies. In: *Proceedings of the 7th Saudi Medical Meeting.* Dammam: King Faisal University, 1982: 248-251.

27. **Shobokshi OA.** Endoscopy of the upper gastrointestinal tract analysis of 551 cases. In: *Proceedings of the 7th Saudi Medical Meeting.* Dammam: King Faisal University, 1980: 879-889.

28. **Amer MH.** Epidemiologic aspects of esophageal cancer in Saudi Arabian patients. *The King Faisal Specialist Hosp Med J* 1985; 5: 69-78.

29. **Monib AEM.** A pilot study of gastrointestinal, pancreatic and liver cancer at King Faisal Hospital, Taif. In: Mahgoub E *et al.* eds. *Proceedings of the 5th Saudi Medical Meeting.* Riyadh: University of Riyadh, 1980: 701-706.

30. **Atiyeh M, Ali MA.** Primary hepatocellular carcinoma in Arabia: a clinical pathological study of 54 cases. *Am J Gastrol* 1980; 74: 25-29.

31. **Blumberg BS, Larouze B, London WT, et al.** The relation of infection with the hepatitis B agent to primary hepatic carcinoma. *Am J Pathol* 1975; 81: 669-682.

32. **Inaba Y, Maruchi N, Matsuda M, et al.** A case-control study on liver cancer with special emphasis on the possible aetiological role of schistosomiasis. *Int J Epidemiol* 1984; 13: 408-412.

33. **Emmons PR, Harrison MJD, Honour AJ, Mitchell JR.** Hepatitis B and hepatocellular carcinoma. *Lancet* 1978; 6: 218.

34. **McMichael AJ.** Oral cancer in the Third World: time for preventive intervention? *Int J Epidemiol* 1984; 13: 403-405.

35. **Hirayama T.** An epidemiological study of oral and pharyngeal cancer in central and south-east Asia. *Bull WHO* 1966; 34: 41-69.

36. **Ibrahim K, Jafarey NA, Zuberi SJ.** Plasma vitamin 'A' and carotene levels in squamous cell carcinoma of the oral cavity and oro-pharynx. *Clin Oncol* 1977; 3: 203-207.

37. **Ernberg N, Kallin B.** Epstein-Barr virus and its association with human malignant diseases. *Cancer Surveys* 1984; 3: 51-89.

38. **Stirling G, Zahran F, Jamjoom A, Eed D.** Cancer of the mouth in the western region of Saudi Arabia: a histopathological and experimental study. *King Abdulaziz Med J* 1981; 1: 10-16.

39. **Amer M, Bull CA, Daouk MN McArthur, P D, Lundmark GJ, El Senoussi M.** Shamma usage and oral cancer in Saudi Arabia. *Ann Saudi Med* 1985; 5: 135-141.

40. **Macaron C, Ali MA, Berghan R.** King Faisal Specialist Hospital experience in thyroid cancer. In: *Proceedings of the 4th Saudi Medical Conference.* Dammam: King Faisal University, 1980: 751-756.

41. **Jamjoom AM.** Two-years' experience in King Abdul Aziz University Hospital, Jeddah, of treatment of advanced cancer of the breast. In: Mahgoub E, *et al.* eds. *Proceedings of the 5th Saudi Medical Meeting.* Riyadh; University of Riyadh, 1980: 619-628.

42. Higgins I. Respiratory disease. In: Last JM, ed. *Maxcy-Rosenau public health and preventive medicine,* 11th ed. New York: Appleton-Century-Crofts, 1980: 1239-1255.

43. **Zahran FM, Baig MHA.** Long term effects of shisha and cigarette smoking on the respiratory system in Saudi Arabia. In: *Proceedings of the 7th Saudi Medical Meeting.* Dammam: King Faisal University, 1982: 160-165.

44. **Snowdon DA, Phillips RL.** Coffee consumption and risk of fatal cancers. *Am J Public Health* 1984; *74:* 820-823.

45. **Mettlin C, Graham S.** Dietary risk factors in human bladder cancer. *Am J Epidemiol* 1979; 110: 255-263.

46. **Anonymous.** Bladder cancer and smoking (Leading article). *Br Med J* 1972; 1:763.

47. **Mee AD.** Aetiological aspects of bladder cancer in urinary bilharzia. *Saudi Med J* 1982; 3: 123-127.

48. **Hicks RM, Walters CL, Elsebai I, El-Aaser** *et al.* Demonstration of nitrosamines in human urine: preliminary observations on a possible etiology for bladder cancer in association with chronic urinary tract infections. *Proc R Soc Med* 1977; 70: 413-7.

49. **Hanash KA, Bissada NK, Abla A** *et al.* Predictive value of excretory urography, ultrasonography, computerized tomography, and liver and bone scan in the staging of bilharzial bladder cancer in Saudi Arabia. *Cancer* 1984; 54: 172-176.

50. **Epstein JH.** *Photocarcinogenesis: a review.* Department of Health, Education and Welfare Publication (NIH) 78-1532, International Conference on Ultraviolet Carcinogenesis. Natl Cancer Inst Monogr 1978; 50: 13-25.

51. **Urbach F.** Welcome and introduction: *Evidence and epidemiology of ultraviolet - induced cancers in man.* International Conference on Ultraviolet Carcinogensis. Natl Cancer Inst Monogr 1978; 50: 5.

52. **Sayigh AAM.** Saudi Arabia and its energy resources. Paper presented at COMPLES Meeting. Dhahran, 1975.

53. **Hannan MA, Paul M, Amer MH, Al-Watban FH.** Study of ultraviolet radiation and genotoxic effects of natural sunlight in

relation to skin cancer in Saudi Arabia. *Cancer Res* 1984; 44: 2192-2197.

54. **Woodhouse NJY. Norton WL.** Low vitamin D levels in Saudi Arabians. *King Faisal Specialist Hosp J* 1982; 2: 127-131.

55. **Sayigh AAM, Sebai ZA, Abdul Halim.** Preliminary study of the solar radiation effect on skin cancer. In: *Proceedings of Biological Society of Saudi Arabia.* Riyadh: University of Riyadh, 1977; 185-200.

56. **Mughal T, Robinson WA.** Malignant melanoma of the skin. *King Faisal Specialist Hosp Med J* 1982; 2: 167-174.

57. **Cardoso E, Sundararajan M.** The naevoid basal cell carcinoma syndrome. *Saudi Med J* 1985; 6: 272-276.

58. **Sabbah R, Schimmelpfenning W, Berry D.** Retinoplastoma in Saudi Arabia. In: *Proceedings of the 4ᵗʰ Saudi Medical Conference.* Dammam: King Faisal University, 1980: 744-750.

59. **Sabbah RS.** Childhood cancer in Saudi Arabia: current problems and suggested solutions. *King Faisal Specialst Hosp Med J* 1982; 2: 273-276.

60. **Rifai S, Aur RJA, Akhtar M. et al.** Malignant small round cell tumor of the thoraco-pulmonary region in childhood. *King Faisal Specialist Hospital Med J* 1985; 5: 127-130.

61. **Bakhsh TM, Mira SA, Serafi AA.** Leiomyosarcoma of the colon. *Saudi Med J* 1985; 6: 454-458.

62. **Bedikian AY, Saleh V, Ibrahim S.** Saudi patients and companions attitudes toward cancer. *King Faisal Specialist Hospital Med J* 1985; 5: 17-25.

63. **Bedikian AY, Saleh V.** An evaluation of the need for psychosocial counselling for Saudi cancer patients. *King Faisal Specialist Hosp Med J* 1985; 5: 91-98.

64. **Bedikian AY, Thompson SE.** Saudi Community Attitude towards Cancer. *Ann Saudi Med* 1985; 5: 161-168.

65. **Kharola AE.** Islamic view of the well-being of man. *J IMA* 1982; 14: 27.

66. **Hanlon JJ, Pickett GE.** *Public health administration and practice.* 8ᵗʰ ed. St Louis: Times Mirror/Mosby, 1984: 3-21.

67. **El Faraidi AH.** Surgical treatment of carcinoma of the oesophagus. *Saudi Med J* 1979; 1: 35-40.

68. **El-Akkad S.** Plans for cancer care in Saudi Arabia (Leading article). *Saudi Med J* 1982; 3: 71-74.

ROAD TRAFFIC INJURIES:

1.   **Punyahotra V.** *Epidemiology of road traffic accidents in Thailand (1980).* National Accident Research Center, National Safety Council of Thailand, 1982.
2.   Anonymous. *Major issues in road traffic safety.* Conference on Road Traffic Accidents in Developing Countries, Mexico City, 9-13 November, 1981. Geneva: World Health Organization.
3.   **Wyatt BG.** The epidemiology of road accidents in Papua New Guinea. *Papua New Guinea Med J* 1980; 23: 60-65.
4.   **Humphries SV.** Seven million casualties. *Central Afr J Med* 1977; 23: 86-88.
5.   **Drury RAB.** The mortality of elderly Ugandan Africans. *Trop Geog Med* 1972; 24: 385-392.
6.   **Baker SP, Sebai ZA, Haddon W.** Injuries due to accidents: an epidemiological study. *J Jordanian Med* 1976; 11: 15-22 (Arabic).
7.   **Wintemute G.** *The size of the problem.* In: *principles for injury prevention in developing countries.* Geneva: World Health Organization, 1985.
8.   *Bayoumi A.* The epidemiology of fatal motor vehicle accidents in Kuwait. *Accidents Analysis and Prevention* 1981; 13: 339-48.
9.   **Weddell JM, McDougall A.** Road traffic injuries in Sharjah. *Int J Epidemiol* 1981; 10: 155-159.
10.   **Eid AM.** Road traffic accidents in Qatar: the size of the problem. *Accidents Analysis and Prevention* 1980; 12: 287-298.
11.   **Ashi JM, El-Desouky M.** *Traffic accidents in the Arab Gulf States.* Secretariat General of Health for the Arab Countries of the Gulf Area, 1981: 99 pp.
12.   **Tamimi TM, Daly M, Bhatty MA, Lutfi AHM.** Causes and types of road injuries in the Asir Province, Saudi Arabia, 1975-1977: preliminary study. *Saudi Med J* 1980; 1: 249-256.
13.   *Anonymous,* Socioeconomic impact of road traffic accidents in Saudi Arabia (editorial). *Saudi Med J* 1980; 1: 246-8.
14.   **Hamour BA.** Epidemiology of road accidents. In: Sebai ZA, ed. *Community Health in Saudi Arabia,* Jeddah: Tihama Publications, 1984: 45-50.

15. **Tawfik OM, Bakhotma MA, Sulaiman SI.** Head injuries in Jeddah — an analytical study of 200 cases. *Saudi Med J* 1985; 6: 25-34.

16. **Khan AA, Mohiuddin MG.** Head injury in Taif — a review of 1,285 cases — a three-year evaluation. In: *Proceedings of the 7th Medical Meeting.* Dammam: King Faisal University, 1982: 669-673.

17. **El-Meshad MH.** Two years' experience in the management of head injuries in Al-Khobar city. In: *Proceedings of the 7th Medical Meeting.* Dammam: King Faisal University, 1982: 674-77.

18. **Khawashki MI, Abdel-Hafez Y, Chabara AR.** Spinal cord injuries. In: Mahgoub ES, ed. *Proceedings of the 5th Medical Meeting.* Riyadh: University of Riyadh, 1981; 589-608.

19. **Al-Saif A.** *System and organization development of traffic administration: theoretical and experimental aspects.* Riyadh: Isha'a Press 1986: 31-39 (Arabic).

20. **Al-Mofarreh MA, Al-Bunyan AM, Ashoor MT, Markakis EJ.** Fatalities in Riyadh Central Hospital with special reference to road traffic accidents. In: *Proceedings of the 8th Saudi Medical Meeting*, Riyadh, 1983: National Guard Medical Department (in press).

21. **Markakis EJ, Youssef A.** RTA injuries as seen in the multiple trauma unit and ICU in Riyadh Central Hospital. In: *Proceedings of the 8th Saudi Medical Meeting*, Riyadh 1983; National Guard Medical Department (in press).

22. **Hamdy MG.** Chest injuries at Riyadh Central Hospital. In: *Proceedings of the 7th Saudi Medical Meeting.* Dammam: King Faisal University, 1982: 710-15.

23. *Ten years traffic accidents 1971-1980.* An official report. Kingdom of Saudi Arabia: General Traffic Department, Public Security. Ministry of Interior.

24. *Carnage on the highways: how U.S. record compares.* US News and World Report, 1981; 78.

25. **Asogwa SE.** Road traffic accidents: the doctor's point of view. *Afr J Med Medical Sci* 1978; 7: 29-35.

26. **Al-Rodhan N, Lifeso RM.** Traffic accidents in Saudi Arabia: an epidemic. (Special communication). *Ann Saudi Med* 1986; 6: 69-70.

27. **Mufti MH.** Road traffic accidents as a public health problem in Riyadh, Saudi Arabia. *J Traffic Med* 1983; 11: 65-9.

28. **Kaprio LA.** Death on the road. *World Health*, October 1975; 4-9.

29. **Levi L.** Autosclerosis. *World Health* 1975: 10-14.

30. **Sabey BE, Grant BE, Hobbs CA.** *Alleviation of injuries by use of seat belts.* Transport and Road Research laboratory Report 1977: SR 289.

31. **Robertson LS.** *Accidents analysis and prevention* 1977; 9: 151.

32. Anonymous. *The highway loss reduction status report.* Washington DC: Insurance Institute for Highway Safety, 1975; 20: 1-8.

33. **Meyer RJ.** Save the child: children and automobile restraints (Editorial). *Am J Pub Hlth* 1981; 71: 122-123.

34. **Scott PP, Barton AJ.** The effects on road accident rates of the fuel shortage of November, 1973 and consequent legislation. Transport and Road Research Laboratory Supplementary Report (United Kingdom) 1976: 239.

35. **Egsmose L. Egsmose T.** Speed limits save lives. *World Health Forum* 1985; 6: 246-247.

36. **Karpf RS, Williams AF.** Teenage drivers and motor vehicle deaths. *Accidents Analysis and Prevention* 1983; 15: 55-63.

37. **Williams AF, Lund AK, Preusser DF.** Driving behavior of licensed and unlicensed teenagers. *J Pub Hlth Policy* 1985; 6: 379-393.

38. **Malaika S.** The value of a trauma center. In: *8th Saudi Medical Conference* Abstracts. Riyadh, Saudi Arabia: Saudi Arabian National Guard, 1983; 89-90.

REFERENCES

Chapter I

HEALTH SERVICES

AN OVERVIEW, PRIMARY HEALTH CARE & HEALTH MANPOWER:

1. *Achievements of the development plans (1970-1985).* Saudi Arabia: Ministry of Planning, 1986; 271 pp.
2. *Kasongo Project Team.* Primary health care for less than a dollar per year. *World Health Forum* 1984; 5: 211-215.
3. *Development of health services and its appropriate manpower* (CK Health Planner). Saudi Arabia: Ministry of Planning, 1984; 386 pp.
4. **Sebai ZA, Miller DL, Ba'aqeel H.** A study of three health centers in rural Saudi Arabia. *Saudi Med J* 1980; 1: 197-202.
5. **Grants JB.** *Situation of children in the world.* UNICEF publication. Oxford: Oxford University Press, 1986: 147-149. (Arabic)
6. *Statistics of children in UNICEF countries.* UNICEF Report. May 1984:214-215.
7. **Girgis TH.** Health statistics advisory service in Saudi Arabia. *WHO Assignment Rep.* EM/ST/125, EM/SAA/HST/001, 1983: 1-2.

8. **Sebai, ZA.** *The Health of the Family in a Changing Arabia: a case study of primary health care.* 3rd ed. Jeddah: Tihama Publications, 1983: 117-128.

9. *World Health Statistical Annual.* Geneva: World Health Organization, 1985: 19-23.

10. **Grants JB.** *Situation of children in the world.* UNICEF publication. Oxford: Oxford University Press, 1985: 120-121. (Arabic)

11. **Searle CM, Gallagher EB.** Manpower issues in Saudi Arabia development. Milbank Memorial Fund Quarterly/*Health and Society* 1983; 61: 659-685.

12. **Sebai ZA.** *The health of the family in changing Arabia: a case study of primary health care.* 3rd ed. Jeddah: Tihama Publications, 1983: 79-80.

13. **Serenius F, Fougerouse D.** Health and nutritional status in rural Saudi Arabia. *Saudi Med J* 1981; 2(Suppl 1): 10-22.

14. *Fourth Development Plan 1985-1990.* Saudi Arabia: Ministry of Planning, 1985: 323-338.

15. International Conference on primary health care, Alma Ata, USSR, September 6-12, 1978. *World Federation of Public Health Association, Conference Bulletin* 1978; 3: 1-2.

16. **Mahler H.** The meaning of health for all by the year 2000. *World Health Forum* 1981; 2: 5-22.

17. **Hellberg H.** Primary Health Care. *World Health Magazine* September 1983: 18-21.

18. **King M.** An Iranian experiment in primary health care: the West Azerbaijan Project. New York: Oxford University Press, 1983: 162-164.

19. **Fisek NH, Erdal Rengin.** Primary health care: a continuous effort. *World Health Forum* 1985; 6: 230-231.

20. **Habicht JP.** *Delivery of primary care by medical auxiliaries: techniques of use and analysis of benefits achieved in some rural villages in Guatemala.* Washington, PAHO, 1973. (PAHO Scientific Publication No. 278.)

21. *Progress in primary health care: a situation report.* Geneva: WHO Publication, 1983.

22. **Mahler H.** Health 2000: the monitoring process has been set in motion. *World Health Forum* 1984; 5: 99-102.

23. *Alma-Ata 1978: Primary health care,* Report of the International Conference on primary health care, Alma Ata, USSR September

6-12, 1978. ("Health for all" series, No. 1) Geneva: World Health Organization, 1978: 50.

24. **Mahler H.** Opening Address. In: *Primary health care - the Chinese experience.* (Report of an Interregional Seminar) Geneva: World Health Organization 1983: 7-8.

25. **Sebai ZA.** *The health of the family in a changing Arabia: a case study of primary health care.* 3rd ed. Jeddah: Tihama Publications, 1983: 117-128.

26. **Sebai ZA.** Primary health care in the district of Al Asiah. In: Sebai ZA, ed. *Community health in Saudi Arabia: a profile of two villages in Qasim region.* 2nd ed. Jeddah: Tihama Publications, 1984: 71-76.

27. **Sebai ZA, Miller DL, Ba'aqeel H.** A study of three health centers in rural Saudi Arabia. *Saudi Med J* 1980; 1: 197-202.

28. *Kuran. Sura V; Maida* (The Table): 2.

29. **Banoub SN.** Primary health care in the Qasim region. In: Sebai ZA, ed. *Community health in Saudi Arabia: a profile of two villages in Qasim region.* 2nd ed. Jeddah: Tihama Publications, 1984: 59-70.

30. **Sebai ZA, El-Hazmi MAF.** Health profile of preschool children in Tamnia villages, Saudi Arabia. *Saudi Med J* 1981; 2(Suppl 1): 68-71.

31. **Beales JG.** Sick health centres and how to make them better. Kent-London: Pitman Medical Publications, 1978: 137-147.

32. **Taylor CA.** Hospitals, primary care and health services research. In: *Proceedings of the role of hospitals in primary health care.* Karachi: Agha Khan Foundation 1981: 1-30.

33. **Oertley R, Hammer TS.** Saudi clinic design benefits patients flow, staff efficiency. *Modern Health Care* 1977; 7: 46-48.

34. **Fulop T, Roemer MI.** *International development of health manpower policy.* WHO Offset Publication No. 61, Geneva: WHO 1982; 149-162. (Arabic)

35. **Eraj YA.** Point of View: Too few doctors in the third world, too many elsewhere. *World Health Forum* 1985; 6: 146-149.

36. **Nutfaji MA.** *Projection of Saudi population by sex and age 1975-2000.* Saudi Arabia: Department of Mathematics and Financial Sciences, Research Center, College of Administrative Sciences, King Saud University 1981; 82 pp. (Arabic)